MW00462120

Octogenarians Say The Darndest Things!

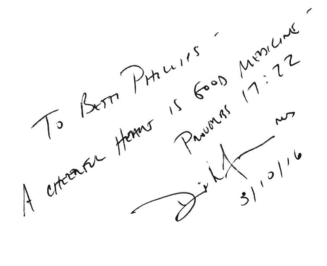

To Betty Phillips -
A cheerful Heart is Good Medicine -
Proverbs 17:22

MD

3/10/16

Also by David L. Anders
You Might Be a Problem Drinker If...
You Might Be a Problem Drinker If...Let's Have Another
Round!
20/80 A Love Letter...Sort Of

Also by Rebekah Yates Anders
The Silver Bell

Octogenarians Say The Darndest Things!

By
David L. Anders, M.D.
with
Rebekah Yates Anders, M.D.

Published in affiliation with David Anders Publishing House
A subsidiary of Anders Peachtree City Properties, LLC
PO Box 2422
Peachtree City, GA 30269
E-mail us at: OctoDoc@AndersUSA.com
Visit our website at: www.AndersUSA.com
Find us on Facebook at David Anders Publishing House

A portion of the earnings from every book sold by
David Anders Publishing House goes to support underprivileged children
in our community.
Find out more at www.AndersUSA.com.

ISBN-13: 978-0615455037 (David Anders Publishing House)

ISBN-10: 0615455034

Cover photo: Gladys Yates and many others

Table of Contents

Dedication by David L. Anders

To Kenya, my wife — on the occasion of her 50th birthday,
Love,
David

*

I wanna grow old with you.
-Adam Sandler

*

Be my life's companion and we'll never grow old.
-The Mills Brothers

*

Dedication by Rebekah Yates Anders

How delightful to be asked by son David to be a consultant for the book he decided to write on aging. I knew a lot about that by virtue of having lived seven dozen years.

Many people are honored by his recollections — family, friends, patients, other writers. All of these are worthy of this dedication.

Even so, I am choosing to dedicate this to BIRTHDAYS. Our family likes to celebrate birthdays, whether in big ways or small. Soon we will celebrate a special person's special birthday, a 50th — a momentous occasion for sure.

Birthdays inspired this book and made it possible. The more birthdays a person has had, the richer the experiences to tell about. God blesses us greatly by letting us live a long time. With His help we can continue to bless others even as age brings many changes.

David and Kenya and their five children have generously shared their home with my husband and me for almost five years. We have been major complications in their busy lives but the whole family treats us like royalty. They take birthdays in stride, even with appreciation and pride.

So, BIRTHDAYS, this dedication is to you, whether one or a hundred and one.

Not to slight fifty. Happy Birthday, Kenya!

The best is yet to be, with God blessing every birthday.

Rebekah Yates Anders

November 13, 2008

*

Grow old along with me! The best is yet to be, the last of life, for which the first was made. Our times are in his hand who saith, 'A whole I planned, youth shows but half; Trust God: See all, nor be afraid!

-Robert Browning (1812-1889)

Acknowledgements
***

As the chief author of this work I have the responsibility of making certain to acknowledge those who made this book possible, so I will start with my mother. Thanks to her for encouraging me to write down the different ways that patients were making my professional life rewarding and memorable. I also thank her for agreeing to serve as a contributor on this project, which unwittingly (on her part) thus committed her to reading and editing the entire book. Her contributions were always of great value, and she did so all the while as continuing her role as wife, mother, grandmother, and Sunday School teacher never missing a beat, and without exposing the surprise gift that this book was intended to be. Thanks also to my wife, Kenya, who having received the text for her birthday, was then able to make helpful and encouraging comments that led to the creation of a book.

Special mention must also be made thanking Mrs. Harry (Mary) Cheves for agreeing with me that it honors the memory of Dr. Harry Cheves to tell his story without concealing his identity. For the same reason I thank Richie Dzio's son, Mr. Henry Vogel, for his approval in telling the story of how Richie blessed my life and so many others.

Finally, I thank all my patients, named or unnamed, who have made my practice of medicine so rewarding with their wit, wisdom, and faith. You inspire me, teach me, humble me, improve me, and prepare me for the next chapters of my life.

Introduction
***

If you ask what is the single most important key to longevity, I would have to say it is avoiding worry, stress and tension. And if you didn't ask me, I'd still have to say it.
- George Burns (1896-1996)

*

(Author's Note to the Reader: If you are looking for the actual things that Octogenarians said and did, skip this introduction and go right to Chapter One. Please do come back and read this introduction at some point, however, because perhaps then the rest of the book will make a little bit more sense. I do know how boring it can be to pick up a book and have to trudge through an introduction that is 2000 words long and has not much to do with the actual reason you picked up the book in the first place. The name of the book is not "How I Came to Write Octogenarians Say The Darndest Things", so I am not surprised if you want to move on. So do I, so let's.)

*

i

Age is not a particularly interesting subject. Anyone can get old.
All you have to do is live long enough.
- Groucho Marx (1890 - 1977)

*

When I was a child growing up in the 1960's, I used to love to watch Art Linkletter's *House Party* on television. One of my favorite portions of the show was when he would interview several children at a time with some fairly ordinary questions and get some fairly extraordinary (or unexpected) answers. This segment, called *Kids Say the Darndest Things* was later revived in a similar format hosted by Bill Cosby, but the kids remained the stars. Even as a child not much older than the children being interviewed, I loved to be surprised by their candid, uninhibited and transparent answers to life's questions.

As a geriatrician for 20 years, I have come to enjoy similar candid, uninhibited, transparent answers that sometimes come from my older patients. Their responses, however, are not rooted in naiveté, but are the results of years of experience and acquired wisdom which they have to share. These experienced seniors are happy to speak up when asked, but they realize that wisdom is best received when volitionally pursued, not forcefully infused. I think many of my patients would agree with Benjamin Franklin who said, "I've had a very happy life. I'd have no objection to living it all over again...But since repetition is impossible, the next best thing is to remember that life and to relate it to others." And relate they will, if we will serve as a receptive audience.

The stereotypical view of the oldest members of our society is that they are a homogeneous group uniformly characterized by slow-witted responses or even dementia, apathy, disability, and uninteresting lives. Far too often the average younger person views the average older person with a bias, an "-ism" that has been called "ageism" by geriatricians. The tottering, demented, out of touch, older person as characterized by Hollywood and drama

ii

does a disservice to the younger and the older alike. Perhaps we all tend to judge elders as a group in part because "they all look the same" or they appear so different from the rest of us. But it is no more fair to accept the senile stereotype than to posit that all adolescents are juvenile delinquents. The term "old" can be used with almost as much negative inflection as to refer to someone as "fat" with the sweeping generalizations that spill over to imply weaknesses in the person's personality and character. Even a child realizes that there are times when calling someone old may not be the most polite way to refer to them, as demonstrated by this conversation with my daughter when she was nine years old: "Dad, when you're *old* like Grandma and Papa...I mean when you're *aged* or *ancient*..."

Life is a continuum, and the elderly are much more like us younger people, often more so than we are comfortable realizing. Yet realize this we must, in order to prepare for the inevitable changes of aging and to better serve those who go before us.

In writing about the great artist it was said: "Since his youth, Rembrandt has had but one vocation: to grow old." In reality, we are all, aware or not, in training for the geriatric years. But how do we prepare? Who will we become? There are numerous books about how to plan for the financial, medical and emotional needs of growing older. But less common are books which allow insight into the actual people that are now older, the people that we will become.

I have come to see that America's elderly are actually a diverse group with some amazing people. After sharing some of their thoughts with you, I think you will agree.

The title of this book, *Octogenarians Say the Darndest Things!*, only begins to tell the story. A better title might be *Octogenarians Do and Say the Darndest, Silliest, Most Profound or Poignant, Funniest, Wisest and Sometimes Profane Things*, but then the spine of the book binding would have to be three feet long, and no library would want to store the book. I also could have used a different decade as the focus of the title, since I've certainly included encounters I've had with patients in their sixties and beyond, but more people seem to know the word "octogenarian" than septuagenarian or nonagenarian, and to use the word "sexagenarian" might raise the prurient interests of an entirely altogether different group of libidinous readers. So I'm sticking with the original title.

While I'm giving explanations of the book itself I should assure you that no patients I've treated are identified by name unless I explicitly state so and have received permission to do so. (Quotes from well-known people who are not my patients are included, but the difference should be obvious.) In some cases I have changed a few demographic facts to respect a patient's privacy. And in some cases I cannot guarantee an exact quote since I wrote the quotes down after leaving the patient's exam room, or later when I arrived home — much later for some, since I did not think to start writing these down until I had been in practice for many years. Some of these events are etched in my memory, and others had to be reconstructed to make my recall fit with the punch-line or the gist of the matter as I could remember it happening. (Can you tell from this paragraph that doctors have become all too familiar with having to give a legal disclaimer for everything they do?) In most cases, the patient's story had nothing to do with why they were in the office that day. Sometimes I'm sure the patient just repeated a story or quote he had already heard, and a few of these quips I've heard from more than one patient or also heard elsewhere, but the tale was delivered with a distinctive quality and in the proper context with impeccable timing. In comedy, timing is everything, so I believe some of these "unoriginals" earn an honorable mention. Remember, I didn't interview anyone for this book. The remarks here were not scripted or prepared. Their spontaneity is part of what makes them notable.

I would like to again thank my mother, who is a retired physician, for agreeing to contribute to this book and serve as my editor and conscience. She knows a lot more about people than I do and can draw on her experience of over fifty years in medicine. I suspect if she didn't have to teach Sunday School next Sunday, she could tell even more memorable stories — or maybe she's holding onto those stories for the sequel to this book. Knowing that she would be reading everything I write has kept me from telling more than I should, for she refines my sensitivity. Physicians as a group have oftentimes developed calluses to some of the social dicta that define what is and is not a proper topic and when or how to discuss such a topic — what other group of people could sit in a hotel banquet hall feasting on a dinner of fine prime rib while watching a PowerPoint presentation on inflammatory bowel surgery? But my mother never developed that callus, or at least never let it affect her behavior, and I am the better for it. And since she is an octogenarian and female, she provides an added dimension that I couldn't otherwise supply. If for some reason you don't like a story here, just remember that she liked it enough to let it go to print, so cut me some slack. Conversely, the story you find you like the most probably came from her.

Finally, before we begin with the entertainment portion of today's program, I would like to thank all the patients who have enriched my life with their style, grace, humor and courage over the years of my practice. I appreciate them entrusting me with their medical care, and the interest they show in my practice, my staff, my family, and my life. They have taught me much, when I was teachable. They have tolerated my human foibles, and occasionally, my comedic foolishness since the first days of my medical practice. Now with a few years behind me, I can better appreciate the observations of Mark Twain: "I was young and foolish then; now I am old and foolisher."

I have provided medical care to people whose faces or accomplishments would make them immediately recognizable to people around the world, and for other people who are equally memorable to me but unknown to most. These patients allow me to reflect on the process of living which is happening all around me, and they have encouraged me to cultivate all the satisfactions possible from life. Sometimes I'm certain it didn't seem like I was fully attentive to their stories as I was also simultaneously attempting to carry out my agenda for their office visit, sorting through a differential diagnosis for their various symptoms to try to deliver the medical care they needed and deserved. I did not want to be too distracted as I thought through which medication or test they would need for sometimes perplexing and troubling situations. Some might be surprised to find I was listening, and listening well.

These vignettes come from the people on the front lines of the battle against growing old too fast, patients and their loved ones. It is never my intention in this book to look like I am poking fun at the older segment of our population. Rather, this is an age we all aspire to become, and yet we younger folks don't really know what to expect. And so I've written this tribute to the determination of the human spirit to see we will all get through this. None of us is going to get out of here alive. As a patient told me, "to live is to age...we all have a terminal condition that is universally fatal: life." But what happens until then? We may try to act brave about growing older, but are we really just whistling at graveyards?

When I first started medical school, my anatomy professor advised our class, "If all the world is a stage, you've just been given a front row seat to the show." Boy, was he right! And what a show it has been. I am much the richer for it, and hopefully after reading what these remarkable people say and do, you will be, too.

*

We don't beat the reaper by living longer, we beat the reaper by living well and living fully.
- Randy Pausch (1960-2008) computer scientist. His "last lecture" about facing terminal pancreatic cancer became an internet sensation and best-selling book.

Wit
***

*

I enjoy seeing the almost lost art form of courtesy and politeness as it is demonstrated in the older generation, particularly those who hail from the long bygone days of the genteel south. One older matron couldn't bring herself to say anything critical about her sister while reporting her family history, so she simply stated, "She was buxom... all over."

*

No matter how old you get, there are parts of the physical exam which remain unpleasant but necessary. One day I had to do a prostate exam on an older gentleman to make certain he wasn't suffering from prostatitis, an infection of the prostate gland. I try to be sympathetic and empathetic to patients undergoing such an exam, and hope to dispel some of their anxieties and discomfort by talking them through the exam, letting them know what to expect, and reassuring them immediately with my findings, especially when my exam reveals a normal, healthy feeling prostate gland. In such an examination the exact feel of the texture, size, symmetry, and firmness of the prostate are all important determinants in disclosing the state of the gland.

Immediately after finishing my exam on this gentleman I tried to assure him by letting him know that nothing had felt abnormal and reported, "That felt good," to which he looked back at me over his shoulder and chuckled, "Speak for yourself, pal."

*

The prostate gland does become the bane of existence for many older men. Not only do men have to worry about developing prostate cancer, but the gland can enlarge, even in the absence of cancer, as a normal of the aging process. This "benign prostatic hypertrophy" can lead to urinary frequency, urgency, and nocturia — having to get up to go to the bathroom at night — symptoms which may make the man more sympathetic for some of the things his wife has been experiencing for years, but symptoms which are otherwise difficult at times for the man to have to discuss with someone else.

As I was reviewing his medical history with an older man who was seeing me for the first time, I asked about some of these urinary symptoms and he shyly responded, "Well, let's just say I now understand why we call them the 'wee hours of the night'."

*

At the risk of going to the well one time too many, here's my last prostate story. I needed to check a man's prostate and was trying to obtain the history to find out the date of his last prostate exam. While flipping through the chart to his previous note, I asked, "Did I do a prostate exam the last time you were here?"

He immediately replied, "No, I'm sure I would have

remembered that. I'm *very* particular about who I let do that to me."

*

An otherwise prim and proper older lady was having to bear with my potentially embarrassing questions as I attempted to determine the cause for her recent onset of diarrhea. When investigating such a problem it can be helpful for the doctor to confirm if there has been any associated bleeding, any fever, the frequency of stool, the amount of stool, etc., etc.

As I was plowing through my questions getting mainly negative responses, I tried to ask about the amount of liquid stool she was producing. I asked, "Has there been a change in the volume of your stools?"

I almost bit through my tongue to keep from laughing when she admitted, "Why yes, they are much louder than they used to be."

*

And while we're on the subject, I might as well tell the story about the man I was interviewing about his recent abdominal pain. "Are you aware of any diarrhea?" I asked. He hurried his answer, demonstrating my questioning was headed in the right direction, "Heck yeah, I'm aware of diarrhea, every time it happens!"

*

Oftentimes patients have to learn a whole new language to be able to best take their medications correctly. In the process of having to take a new pill, they may become acquainted with the name of a diagnosis ("GastroEsophageal Reflux Disease, or

3

"GERD"), a class of drugs (antacids "Proton Pump Inhibitors, or "PPIs"), a generic name ("esomeprazole magnesium"), and a brand name ("Nexium"). Or they may just settle for knowing they take "a purple pill".

Sometimes the information I receive from the patient is packaged even more creatively, such as the time I was asking a man if he was taking his antacid. He looked to his daughter for help in knowing which medication I was talking about. She responded, "Yes, he's taking it," and then, looking toward her father, she said, "You know, your 'Bob Barker' pill." I chuckled at the name given the pill, and didn't recall hearing that Bob Barker was endorsing any specific medication, so I couldn't resist asking why this pill was now so named. I learned a new trick when he replied, "We take the aspirin and blood pressure pill every morning at breakfast, and the purple pill every morning when Bob Barker comes on."

*

The marketing of medications has changed an awful lot during the lifetime of my older patients. But at least some of them seem to be aware that the slick advertising now seen on television on a daily basis is designed to make them want to purchase the newer but more expensive medications.

"You know, Dr. Anders, I think I've just about figured out this drug company thing. They put a lot of commercials on TV just so you'll want to go out and buy their drug. Why, I saw a commercial the other day — a beautiful woman and a man on a beach. They were riding a horse. Looked like they were having a wonderful time. And the medicine they were selling was for a ... social disease. Heck, it made me want to go out and get infected just so I could have as much fun as they were having."

*

4

Internet abbreviations are well known, including the letters "LOL" to represent "Laughing Out Loud", but when I was receiving my medical training in the 1980's before the days of the internet, "LOL" was an abbreviation for "Little Old Lady". Almost every day I see why the two are easily interchangeable. A seemingly prim and proper "LOL" was undergoing a breast exam, during which she tried to break the ice by explaining, "Doctor, I've gone from being a 34-C to being a 38-Long!"

*

Mrs. Bender had returned for a follow-up appointment after I sent her for a liver scan. She was now waiting in the exam room for the results of her test. Unfortunately, I had not yet received a copy of her report. My staff scurried around, calling the radiology department to see if a copy could be faxed over so we could continue with Mrs. Bender. I decided to go on in to the exam room and see Mrs. Bender to address any other problems as we waited to hear about her report, hoping that perhaps she had heard directly from the radiology department regarding her liver test after the scan had been read by the radiologist.

"Mrs. Bender, was your liver read?" I asked.

"I don't know," she replied. "What color was it supposed to be?"

*

Mr. Johns was a man who had worked all his life, hard. He was now well over 70, and still quite an impressive physical specimen. All six feet five inches of his height nicely distributed the 280 pounds on his frame which seemed to be mostly muscle. But arthritis was encroaching at an increasing pace — his hips, knees, hands, elbows, shoulders, and lower back all ached from the years of manual labor that he had performed. He realized this was, in part, a price of the years of work he had demanded of his body, and he didn't complain as much about it as most would. But he did confide to me one day, "Doc, whoever said that 'hard work never hurt anybody' never did any hard work!"

*

Mr. Pickens was a man who lived life on his own terms. He had survived to the age of 80 years despite being grossly overweight, and he wasn't about to be changed by any preaching I could deliver about proper dieting.

"Dr. Anders, I want you to understand, I *love* good food. I eat whatever I want to eat, whenever I want to eat, wherever I want to eat. I'm enjoying spending my money, lots of it, on food." Patting either side of his considerable girth, he continued, "They say you can't take it with you, but I'm certainly going to try!"

*

Georgia can be hot in the summertime, and no one who grew up in Georgia in the days before air-conditioned homes has forgotten what summer in Georgia used to be like. When I was evaluating a patient one day we reviewed his prior exposure to toxins, and he recalled the days many years ago when his family would vacation on the Georgia coast during the summer to try to escape some of the inland heat. Unfortunately, when visiting the coast in that day one traded problems with mosquitoes for the heat. He recalled playing outside while the city trucks drove by spraying out a fine mist of "mosquito poison", and he still wonders just what he may have been exposed to. In typical good fashion, he shrugged it off — he has lived as long as he thought he would, and outlived his wife. But he couldn't resist entertaining me with

6

a tall tale about how big the mosquitoes could grow along the coast:

Two mosquitoes were hovering over their victim, just about to make an attack. "Should we eat him here or take him home?" asked the first.

"We'd better eat him here," said the second mosquito. "If we take him home, the big guys will take him away from us."

*

As I walked into the examining room I could see a look of exasperation on Mr. Jacob's face and knew that a flare of his arthritic knees was likely. He nevertheless began the conversation with a good natured complaint: "Doc, getting old is getting old!"

*

Knees do seem to be the source of pain and concern for many older patients. Arthritis is one of the top reasons older patients go to see a doctor, and patients and doctors alike look forward to the day that better treatment and even cures are available. Until then, we physicians should continue to do all we can to bring relief, realizing this is no trivial issue for patients. Too often patients, family members, and doctors blame a variety of symptoms on "old age", and put off concerns of real disease as simply being the unavoidable consequences of a long life. Fortunately for me, early in my career a patient taught me what not to say, even before I said it, although I'm sure I must have thought it, when he told me the following story.

An eighty-year-old man went to the doctor to see why his right knee caused him so much trouble. The doctor examined his knee, and having established the diagnosis of osteoarthritis, tried to reassure the patient. His reassurance came across as

7

condescending, as he told the patient, "You have to expect some of these things; don't forget this knee is 80 years old." The pained patient, hoping for a better answer or at least a treatment for pain, rolled up his left pants leg, pointed at his other knee, and exclaimed, "Well, Doc, this knee is 80 years old, too, and it doesn't give me a bit of trouble!"

*

My last patient of the day was new to me. Mr. Jenkins was 76, healthy, still working in the retail sales company he owned, and was seeing me only because he wanted a screening medical exam. His engaging personality confirmed that he should have a natural talent in selling to others, and I enjoyed getting to know him as we talked about his life and health. As I was summarizing my findings with him, he got a twinkle in his eye and said, "Doc, your staff told me I was your last patient for the day, and I appreciate you not rushing through my appointment so you could leave. So now I'll tell you my forecast. I think I'm going to live to be 152."

Oftentimes a patient will tell me he expects to live to be 100 since one or more of his ancestors did, but never before had anyone been quite this optimistic. So I had to bite on his set-up and ask just how this could be possible.

"Well," he continued, enjoying an audience, "I'm 76, and I feel half dead!"

*

And then there was Mrs. Cox who was feeling every one of her 81 years. "I was doing fine until I hit 80, and then it hit back!"

*

8

I was seeing Mr. Jefferson for the first time. He had a weathered and worn appearance, looking even older than his 82 years, if such a thing is possible. Something he said implied he had lived in our community since his childhood, which meant he would likely have grown up farming the poor dirt soil of the depression.

Hoping to hear something about how Fayette County was before the current influx of Volvos and BMWs filled so many new subdivisions, I asked, "Have you lived here all your life?"

"All my life's not up yet," he volleyed back.

*

I take it as a good sign when I meet an older patient who is trying to stay young, trying to look younger. Doing so seems to keep people more plugged-in to life. One of my older men joked about such efforts as they related to impressing the fairer sex.

"Two well-to-do gentlemen who were over seventy were talking at the country club. The first was bragging about the beautiful 30-year –old woman he had just married. "Wow!" said the second man when he saw her picture, "How did you get her to marry you?"

"I lied about my age," replied the first.

"Did you tell her you were fifty?" asked the second man.

"Nope, I told her I was ninety."

*

Vanity persists into the eighties and beyond. I see that as a good indicator — of a person who still wants to be respected and accepted by others. It may surprise you to find that despite the wrinkles, stooped shoulders, thinning and gray hair, and slowed gait that identify them as "senior", more than one elderly lady (and even an occasional man) has admitted, often after the tattling of a

9

son or daughter, that they don't want to use a cane . When I ask why, inevitably the answer seems to be that, "someone will think I am old."

I have learned not to argue in such a situation, but to try to point out the danger they place themselves in when they risk stumbling. Any fall could have catastrophic consequences and life changing results. I encourage them not to worry about what others are thinking, reminding them that "Pride goeth before a fall."

*

I was seeing Mrs. Martin again with her daughter accompanying her. We were reviewing her symptoms and interval history, and I asked if she was using her walking cane to help prevent falls. Her daughter assured me that she always used her cane or that an appointed friend or family member was walking right beside her. "We are very careful now, and she always has her cane, or uses a designated walker."

*

Getting old is something that comes naturally, but not easily. Many patients have warned me that "getting old is not for sissies". A more novel expression of a similar sentiment came from the woman who told me, "I'm a tough old bird. But aging is quite a meat tenderizer."

*

One of my older ladies is actually quite independent and healthy at the age of 84. But even she has noted some changes over the years, and notes with a chuckle that for her, "Old age is just one humiliation after another."

*

I should learn to expect the unexpected when I talk with patients. But I keep getting surprised. I went in to check a patient returning for follow-up to see how her change in medications was improving her blood pressure. I asked, "How do you feel?" to which she deadpanned, "With my hands."

*

To continue in that vein, I was seeing a 91-year-old woman with her daughter. The woman was having some problems with irritability. I wanted to make certain she was getting enough sleep, so I asked her, "How do you sleep?" to which she snapped back, "With my eyes closed!"

*

Dr. Ike Reighard (who is not yet elderly) was my pastor for most of the second twenty years of my life. He performed my wedding and has been more than just a pastor to me and my family. As he relates in his book *Treasures From the Dark* my mother served as his obstetrician, but that's another story — get the book!

Since I was his doctor for several years, I can include the following as "something a patient gave me", even though he read the poem, "My Younger Days", by Maya Angelou to me and hundreds of others during a sermon he delivered one Sunday when he returned to my home church. It concludes with the thought:

Though my hair has turned to gray
And my skin no longer fits,
On the inside, I'm the same old me,
It's the outside that has changed a bit.

*

Another story that is not from a patient but deserves mention is the conversation I heard between two older patrons of the Atlanta Symphony Orchestra when I was at a concert not long ago. One gentleman told the other, "Yesterday I went to the neuro-physiatrist to relieve a pain I got the day before when I was being treated by the physical therapist."

*

Sometimes there is no substitute for patience when trying to understand what someone, especially an older someone, is trying to tell you. Especially in the practice of medicine, where in medical school doctors are taught that "the history is 85% of the diagnosis", which means that often times listening to the patient is more important than examining the patient if the doctor wants to get a good idea of what is going on. And try though you may, as a physician, you will never be able to listen faster than the patient can speak. If that patient speaks slowly, you had better pull up a chair.

One such experience I had was with an older man whose name is long forgotten, but his story remains as fresh in my memory as ever. I was a first year, wet-behind-the-ears, over-worked and under-slept intern at the Medical College of Georgia, doing a six-week rotation on the Internal Medicine service at the Veteran's Affairs (V.A.) Medical Center inpatient service. As such I would get called down to the emergency room to evaluate patients who were sick enough to be considered for admission.

One night when I had already been awake 20 hours and knew I had another 16 hours before I could leave the hospital, I was called down to evaluate an older man who was having gastroenteritis.

He was a retired man whose speech revealed not much education, but his smile revealed a very human heart. Despite his misfortune at the time, he seemed to be in a better mood than I was. I was hoping that his case would be straightforward enough so that he could go home and I could grab a nap before the next patient came in. But he was in no rush. Every question I asked was followed by a long pause, a stroke of his stubbly chin, an upward rolling of the eyes, and then an answer that was often less helpful than it was long. He seemed to think I was a lawyer taking a deposition and that every question I presented was craftily structured to catch him in an inconsistency, so he was obligated to evaluate every possible angle before responding. Like Sergeant Joe Friday of Dragnet, I wanted to scream "Just the facts!" but I knew that wouldn't get me anywhere. Nevertheless, when asked a simple straightforward question such as, "Have you had any fever?" I had hoped that the answer — "yes" or "no" — would be contained within the first few words out of his mouth. I realized that was not happening.

In gastroenteritis, there are many questions that should be asked, and I was dutifully doing so, learning oh so much about his neighbors, his family, his past work experience, his philosophy on the V.A. medical system, his previous war experience, his wife's family, his son's neighbors, his daughter's past work experience, his barber's philosophy on the V.A. medical system, — you get the picture. Not that I asked, it just seemed an important part of the story to him. I would try to redirect the question when possible, but his slow, halting speech never allowed me to be sure that I wasn't just about to cut him off as he was going to give the answer I so yearned for.

One of the questions to be asked was what food he had eaten recently, to know if food poisoning should be a consideration for the differential diagnosis. So I interrupted his drawn-out recounting of the successes and failures of the Roosevelt Works Progress Administration to blurt out, somewhat curtly, "What did you eat this morning?"

My change in tone seemed to capture his attention, and I was momentarily hopeful that my newfound assertiveness would help keep him on track and answering the questions more directly. He leaned back in his chair and started, "Well, let's see..." (stroking the chin), "... I had, um... um... ummm," (narrowing his eyes and rolling them back upward and to the left), "this morning...hmmm..." (now slowly rolling frontward and backward in his chair with a mesmerizing rhythm that set me swaying in sympathetic harmonic motion so as to encourage this revelation), "this morning I had.. I ate... breakfast!"

*

I'm a great proponent of multi-generational families. I realize every situation is different, but when the personalities, finances, health status, and mental health are properly aligned, the richness of life's experiences is multiplied with the presence of another generation in the household. Admittedly, this must require a good bit of adjustment and personal sacrifice on the part of each generation involved.

I was inquiring just how such an arrangement was going with an active and dynamic 83-year-old woman who is in my practice. I recalled that she lived in a household that consisted also of her daughter, her single mom granddaughter, and newly arrived great-granddaughter. They all live together in one house, HER house, as the other family members have moved in with her. She now had plenty of opportunities to cook, clean, and babysit. She seemed proud of the fact that she still lived in her own house, noting, "all of my friends are now living in assisted living". The thought gave her pause, then she laughed and said, "Come to think of it, I live in assisted living too, but I'm the one providing all the assistance."

14

*

Mr. Chastain is the kind of geriatric patient I enjoy treating. Completely independent at the age of 82 he still enjoys doing his own yard work and participating in his church choir. Although widowed three years ago, he is upbeat and brings a smile to my face just by having his name on my daily printed schedule. The honor of being entrusted with his medical care is enhanced by the fact that I went to school with his son 30 years ago, and while his son has moved out of state, I keep up with him via his dad.

One day I walked into the exam room with Mr. Chastain, my words of apology almost preceding me into the room as I expressed regret for being 30 minutes behind schedule and for keeping him waiting. As I raised my penitent head for the first actual eye contact after the compact confession that had lasted precisely long enough to allow me to take my seat on my stool, I could see the sparkle in his eye that told me I would finish his appointment even further behind in the day's schedule.

"Up until last week I was ready to come back here today and really let you have it. That new cholesterol pill you put me on last visit really threw me for a loop. Two weeks after you started me on it I started having trouble sleeping, my throat felt sore, and I just didn't feel like me. I was sure it was all because of that new medicine, and I was just about to throw those samples in the trash. But then last week everything went back to normal and I'm still on the medicine and I feel great, so I don't think it's fair to blame the pills. I guess I was just a little anxious about being on a new medicine. But it taught me an important lesson about life," he said, uninterrupted.

"What's that?" I asked, only temporarily halting his soliloquy, as if he wouldn't continue without my prompting.

"A man should always have a wife, a dog, and be on at least one medication, so there will always be something to blame anything on."

Mr. Baker was a soft-spoken, no non-sense kind of man who was approaching his 85th birthday. I asked if he had any plans to make the day memorable. He acted as if he didn't think there was much special about turning 85 years old, but I responded that to do so was quite a milestone in life. He shrugged, and then conceded, "I guess a milestone is better than a tombstone."

I had a friend who had just turned 55 years old, and so I shared the "better a milestone than a tombstone" quote with him. He replied that he had teased his father about celebrating yet another birthday, but his father assured him that he "would far rather be seen than viewed."

And I think it was Art Linkletter who said, "It's better to be over the hill than under it."

We all sometimes forget that words and phrases don't always have the same meaning to all people. I was discussing the cost of medications with a patient and trying to express my realization that expenses can be tight when living on a fixed income. He interrupted me to say, "Heck, my income's not fixed, it's broken!"

The transition into retirement can be a challenge. A woman I was treating hinted at as much one day as she reflected how her life had changed when her husband retired. "Suddenly I had half as much income and twice as much husband!"

*

Another patient bragged about how great retirement was for him: "The week-end starts on Monday!"

*

Mrs. Rivers was a well-established patient who had been in my practice for several years, a friend of my mother-in-law who had first come to see me shortly after her husband died. Her days are now filled with time spent with her son and her grandchildren. One day, seemingly for no reason, she told me that a high school classmate had contacted her to ask her out for a date. I asked her if she took him up on his offer, and she laughed and said, "No, I didn't find him attractive in high school, why would I start now?" She then confided that there was one classmate she knew of whom she would be very interested, but that he was married, so she wouldn't pursue him. She implied the choices for a soon to be eighty-year-old woman were fairly limited, and that her friends had advised her to proceed with caution. "They tell me that at age, all that men want are a nurse, a purse, or worse..."

*

Another woman confided in me to report that sometimes it was not easy to meet a desirable man at her advanced age. She joked that one of her friends had advised her, "At our age, finding a good man is like trying to find a parking space at Wal-Mart. All

17

the good ones are already taken, and if you do think you've found a good one, it turns out to be handicapped."

*

Sometimes people bring me in things they have seen elsewhere, spam e-mails with jokes about medicine and health, newspaper articles about the latest new treatment, magazine articles about vitamins, etc. One of the things I kept was given to me by a woman who was getting older, but could find the humor in her situation. She seemed to embody the adage, "He who laughs, lasts." I don't know who the author was, but the original title on the sheet she gave me was "How to Know You're Growing Older." In my mind, this might be even funnier if you use your imagination to hear Jeff Foxworthy proclaiming, "You *might* be growing older if...":

- Everything hurts and what doesn't hurt, doesn't work.
- The gleam in your eyes is from the sun hitting your bifocals.
- You feel like the night after, and you haven't been anywhere.
- Your little black book contains only names ending in M.D.
- You get winded playing chess.
- Your children begin to look middle-aged.
- You finally reach the top of the ladder and find it leaning against the wrong wall.
- You join a health club and don't go.
- You decide to procrastinate, but then never get around to it.
- You're still chasing women but can't remember why.
- Your mind makes contracts your body can't meet.
- A dripping faucet causes an uncontrollable bladder urge.

- You know all the answers, but nobody asks you the questions.
- You look forward to a dull evening.
- You walk with your head high trying to get used to your bifocals.
- Your favorite part of the newspaper is "25 Years Ago Today..."
- You turn out the light for economic rather than romantic reasons.
- You sit in a rocking chair and can't make it go.
- Your knees buckle and your belt won't.
- You regret all those mistakes resisting temptation.
- You're 17 around the neck, 42 around the waist, and 96 around the golf course.
- You stop looking forward to your next birthday.
- After painting the town red, you have to take a long rest before applying a second coat.
- You're startled the first time you are addressed as an old timer.
- You remember today, that yesterday was your anniversary.
- You just can't stand people who are intolerant.
- The best part of your day is over when your alarm clock goes off.
- You burn the midnight oil until 9 pm.
- Your back goes out more often than you do.
- A fortune teller offers to read your face.
- Your pacemaker makes the garage door go up when you watch a pretty girl go by.
- The little gray-haired lady you help across the street is your wife.
- You have too much room in the house and not enough room in the medicine cabinet.
- You sink your teeth into a steak and they stay there.

Mrs. Warren had reached 92 years of age almost unscathed, until she took quite a tumble while on vacation. Fortunately, no bones were found to be broken when she was examined in the emergency room, but when she returned to town she came into the office for an exam just to be sure everything was OK. I could tell just by looking at her that she was having significant pain, fractures or no, and several deep bruises confirmed her story. As she winced with each move I tried to convey my sympathy for her painful situation. Her lifelong optimism rose to the surface though, as she advised me, "I'll be OK; I understand the first hundred years are the hardest."

*

Mr. Lloyd was another great example of playing the hand life has dealt. The aches and pains of aging were catching up with him, and everything seemed to be wearing out at once, but he wasn't going to complain. However, with his dry humor he could not help but observe, "Unfortunately, my body only has a lifetime warranty. I wish I could have gotten a longer one."

*

Two doctors were attending a conference on geriatrics at a large downtown hotel. During the afternoon break they decided to go outside for a brief walk to stretch their legs. As they walked, they discussed some of the points from an earlier lecture, including the theoretical maximum age of a human being. Each remarked on having taken care of patients over the age of one hundred years. While they were talking they walked past a coffee shop, inside of which sat a man they both agreed appeared to be the oldest man they had ever seen. Emboldened by the research reports they had heard that day, they decided to step inside and talk with the gentleman and find out his secrets for longevity. After brief introductions and an explanation, the man slowly and meticulously began to outline his pathway to getting as old as he was:

"Well, I've lived a pretty wild life, gone through five wives, sleep very little, and drink lots of coffee. Every day I drink a fifth of bourbon. I smoke at least a pack of cigarettes each day, and I've never exercised a day in my life."

"Wow!" exclaimed the first doctor. "And just how old are you?" he asked.

To which the man replied proudly, "I'm 57 years old."

*

In the words of Bill Cosby, "I told you that one so I could tell you this." And this one is a true story.

Every summer our family vacations at Daytona Beach, Florida. One of my pleasures is to get up early and go for a 5 mile walk on the beach before the sun becomes too hot. Recently my teenaged daughter, Rebekah, has joined me. It is a great opportunity for us to discuss a myriad of things, including health, fitness and longevity while we walk on one of the world's most beautiful wide beaches and take in the sites of whatever may have washed up on the beach overnight, watch the sun rise, and see hundreds of other walkers and joggers of every age, shape and size.

One morning we saw going the opposite direction a healthy appearing senior citizen who I guessed to be well past eighty years old. After we got past her I commented to Rebekah on what amazingly good posture, steady gait that required no cane, and toned legs the lady had, despite her apparent age. The next morning we saw the same lady walking toward us again. I could not resist the urge to know more about her, so I politely approached her and introduced myself and my daughter.

"I'm a doctor and I treat a number of people who are doing a great job of taking care of themselves. We saw you out walking here yesterday and again today and, if you'll forgive me, I wanted to ask, how old are you?"

Her quick eyes and gentle smile revealed a very alert lady. Her answer impressed this middle-aged dad and his teen daughter: "I retired down here from the Northeast, and live a few miles over. I drive here to the beach when the weather is good and take a morning walk. And I just turned 90 a few days ago."

*

I have a dear little lady for a patient who has figured out the real way to lose weight. "Doctor, I've finally found the diet that works. It is called 'The Nancy Reagan Diet'. You 'Just Say No' to everything!"

*

"Doctor Anders, I've thought about what you told me at the last visit," my somewhat talkative and recently turned 70 patient said, "about what I can try to do to live to be 100 years old. And with all the things you suggested I quit doing, start doing, do more of, and do less of, I decided that even if I didn't live 100 years, it would certainly seem that long."

*

My older patients are often accompanied by their children, or children-in-law. The children are sometimes embarrassed by their parents' actions in my presence, although I'm actually pretty hard to surprise. I was caught off guard one day by the exchange between a somewhat exasperated daughter and her jovial father:

"Now Dad, we need to be respectful of Doctor's time and settle down for just a minute. Can't you act your age?"

"Kittie, if I acted my age, I'd have rigor mortis."

*

A similar refrain was heard on another day by a patient who had recently celebrated another birthday. He asked: "Do you realize that the average person my age is dead?"

*

And to round out this trio of morbid thoughts: I will occasionally feel comfortable enough in my relationship with an older patient to be able to reassure them that, "You will not die prematurely."

*

Some folks seem to age more gracefully than others, accepting the changes of the seasons of life as they approach. It can be entertaining to watch someone else try to hold onto the last remnants of their youth long after the rest of the world realizes that time has passed. One patient laughed at her own denial towards aging when she saw the following, so she gave me a copy:

Things Are Changing
- Everything is farther away now than it used to be. It's twice as far to the corner and they have added a hill, I notice.
- I have given up running for the bus, it leaves faster than it used to.
- It seems to me they are making steps steeper than in the old days.

- And have you noticed the smaller print they use in the newspapers?
- There is no sense in asking anyone to read aloud. Everyone speaks in such a low voice that I can hardly hear them.
- The material in clothing is getting very skimpy, especially around the waist and the hips.
- It's almost impossible to reach my shoe laces now.
- Even people are changing. They are so much younger than they used to be when I was at their age.
- On the other hand people my age are so much older than I am.
- I ran into an old friend the other day and she had aged so much she didn't recognize me.
- I got to thinking about the poor thing while I was combing my hair this morning. In doing so, I glanced at my reflection, and confound it, they don't even make good mirrors like they used to.

*

My mother's Aunt Dorothy used to recite a poem she had learned about this same denial:

> *My face in the mirror*
> *isn't wrinkled or drawn.*
> *My furniture's dusted,*
> *the cobwebs are gone.*
> *My garden is lovely*
> *and so is the lawn.*
> *Don't think I'll ever put*
> *my glasses back on!*

*

A woman well into her 80's brought her husband in to see me because he had slowed considerably during the past few weeks. She was concerned that he might have an underlying condition beyond natural aging that might be going undiagnosed. She was visibly concerned about her spouse, but still found humor in her situation. "He's acting like the old man in the joke where the wife asked her husband, 'What are you going to do today?' and the husband replies, 'Nothing.' The wife says back to the husband, 'but you did that yesterday', and the husband says, 'but I didn't finish!'"

*

Like most doctors, I find my daily patient schedule is dominated by the unexpected at times. Often when one patient suffers (and I have to focus an unplanned extra amount of time and attention on that patient), all patients suffer (by having to wait longer to see me than they or I wish they had to). I am almost unfailingly impressed by how understanding and accommodating other patients are in this situation, but sometimes the patient does have his say. Like the time I was late seeing Mr. McCartney. As I entered the room with my apologies to him and his wife, he said, "That's OK, but can you tell me where I can get a good haircut?"

Hoping this odd start was a joke, I decided to play straight man to his inquiry and simply stated that Randy down the road was who cut my hair, vainly realizing as I responded that maybe he was actually envying my hair. I was quickly put back in my place when his own Gracie Allen of almost sixty years then interjected, "Well, old man, why didn't you get a haircut before you came in here?"

To which he could then retort, "Because I didn't need a haircut when I came in!"

*

And another story on being untimely: as I entered the room behind schedule, Mr. Hills said "Oh, so you're not dead after all?" I started in with, "I am sorry for keeping you waiting—" to which he interrupted with, "Oh, I don't mind. It's just that in the waiting room I heard two women talking and one referred to you as 'The Late Dr. Anders'".

*

And then again, sometimes I'm behind schedule, not because I'm slow, but because (it might seem to you), the patient is slow. Yes, sometimes it does take longer to get a history from an older patient, and yes, sometimes they might speak a little slower or take a little longer moving from "Point A" to "Point B". (Incidentally, to the frustration of all doctors, Medicare doesn't seem to understand this, and expects physicians to bill an otherwise healthy thirty-year-old patient with two or three problems the exact same fee as a ninety-year-old patient with a list of ten medications, multiple problems, and who is rightly deserving of additional time. Medicare tells us physicians we can give all the time we want...we just can't bill for it! Of course, knowing the rules for billing Medicare is all a bit more complicated than that so many physicians just don't accept Medicare, but I digress...).

Nevertheless, sometimes the patient is slow, but when I'm 90 years old, I'm going to be taking a little extra time to smell the roses, too! Hurrying in an unfamiliar environment can be dangerous and lead to falls, so I do not want my older patients who are at an increased risk of falling to feel pressured to hurry while in my office. The patients usually understand and appreciate my approach, but sometimes they seem a little self-conscious nevertheless. They usually do not want to be slow any more than you or I. One day, as I was cautiously helping Mrs. Wall onto the examination table I reminded her, "Now take your time."

Her insightful response reminded me of just how aware she was of her time and my time: "Doctor, I'm sorry I'm old and slow. I think you should say, 'Now take *my* time!' But thank you for taking the time to keep me safe."

*

I suppose I could lie and say this happened to me but since a patient told this story to me, repeating this is in keeping with the theme of this book.

A man who was very hard of hearing finally broke down and purchased a hearing aid. Not just any aid would do — he had to have the best. He wound up with a digital audio, remote control, super small, high fidelity, dual frequency, miniaturized hearing aid. He couldn't wait to show it off to his family and friends.

"Let me show you my new hearing aid, since I'm sure you wouldn't notice it yourself," he told his best friend as they started a golf date.

"What's so special about it?" asked his friend.

"It is a digital audio, remote control, super small, high fidelity, dual frequency hearing aid, and it cost me over ten thousand dollars, but it is worth it!" proclaimed the proud owner with glee.

"Wow!" exclaimed his friend, thinking he might need one someday, "what kind is it?"

The man glanced at his wrist and replied, "Almost two o'clock."

*

And the other hearing aid story I heard that bears repeating was of a wealthy but eccentric man who was incredibly hard of hearing but refused to get a hearing aid. His family took him to the doctor on several occasions specifically to undergo hearing testing and get hearing aids, but the man persistently refused to get hearing aids, despite testing which confirmed profound hearing loss. The frustration of the family members was obvious, as they stood directly in front of the man, face to face, shouting for him to hear, or perhaps just read their lips, and sometimes resorting to writing things down so he could understand them.

Then one day he showed up at the doctor's office and the doctor immediately noticed quite a difference. The man could hear. The doctor asked him and the man proudly reported, "I finally visited the Mayo clinic and was fitted with a new type of hearing aid that is practically invisible, doesn't have to be removed, and is painless for the wearer, but works great!"

Knowing how relieved the family must be to finally be able to communicate without shouting, the doctor inquired to what their response had been.

"Oh, I haven't told them yet. But I have already changed my will three times!"

*

Over the years I have been fortunate to have been trusted by dozens of ministers to provide their medical care. I admire the examples of grace and patience I have seen in most of them, and they don't usually complain about very much, having learned over the years to tolerate the failings that characterize us as humans.

A retired pastor and I were discussing his new schedule and I was surprised to hear how often he was still called on to conduct weddings and funerals, for which I surmised he did not receive fair pay on some occasions. "Well, you know what they say about preachers," I said, "you don't ever retire, you just stop getting paid." To which he responded, "I thought it was 'Old preachers never retire, they just get put out to pastor.'"

*

I've only got one wrinkle and I'm sitting on it.
- Jeanne Calment, "The World's Oldest Person" (1875-1997)

Wisdom
***

Is not wisdom found among the aged? Does not long life bring understanding?
- Job 12:12 (NIV)

*

The first time I met Frank Fenton Forth, Jr. his passion and enthusiasm for life were quite evident. "Call me 'Frank', you must call me 'Frank'", he said brightly as he shook my hand. While well past 80 years old, he energized me just by being in his presence. On a subsequent visit he gave me a copy of the book he had written about his life as a forester and his love for his wife and children. The book was published when Frank was 84. In the Foreword of *The Forester's Notebook* he writes about the span of his life and summarizes his philosophy on living a long, productive life: "1923-2??? It's really the <u>dash</u> that's important."

*

Mrs. Lucas was an interesting little lady who grew up in a small town in southern Georgia. The people there had been close, and she still enjoyed returning to her hometown to see longstanding friends. On a recent trip her family took her around to visit friends, and friends' grave sites. At the age of 88, she was reflective on how much things had changed, on how she was the only one from her high school class who was still fairly independent. She seemed particularly moved to realize how infirm and disabled one of her classmates now was. "He was the fastest one in the class — basketball, football, he could do it all. Now he is an invalid."

She paused, then continued, "Being the last one standing seems like a good goal. We all want to live a long time, if we can do so in good health. There is a price to be paid for longevity, and that is having to watch all those you know and love suffer and die... I'm now the best athlete in my class."

*

I knew Mr. Powell, now retired, had made a lot of money in the residential real estate market. He was still fit and active. I was impressed by his health as to how well he had taken care of his body and after examining him, I told him so. I knew exactly what he meant when he replied, "Too many people treat their bodies like renters, not owners."

*

Mrs. James was a very pleasant widow who seemed to be the envy of anyone her age, and probably many people younger. She was well past 80, energetic, enthusiastic, and a quick conversationalist. She had made some concessions to age — she no longer drove her car, and arthritic knees limited her mobility. I asked her why she always seemed so optimistic, and was impressed with her reply:

"If we only focus on what we can no longer do, on what we don't have, we will be very

disappointed. I have friends who keep themselves miserable doing just that. But, if we only focus on what we *do* have, what we *can* enjoy, who we *do* know, we will be very thankful, indeed."

*

Turning ninety years old is a lifetime accomplishment which very few people actually achieve. I enjoy interacting with these folks, realizing they all have a story to tell, much wisdom to impart, and a little more to do before their time is up. Most ninety-year-old people seem to be surprised how quickly life happened, and can yield good advice if we slow down long enough to take the time to listen. On many patient visits I have not had a whole lot to offer to change the challenges and struggles that face the most elderly, but I do try to remember to let them make me better by hearing what they have to say.

One such woman seemed ready to impart advice one day, and so I listened. "Ninety seems to be the breaking point. After that, everything goes wrong," she said, with a smile fueled by gratefulness, not regret.

*

I was seeing Mrs. Aaron for the first time since her ninetieth birthday. I congratulated her and inquired about how she had celebrated. She reported she was still basking in the glow of a big party her family had given her, so I asked her, "What's the best part about turning 90?" Neither her daughter nor I expected her immediate enthusiastic answer, "The liquor!" As I laughed while trying to figure out where to go from there, she went on, "Doctor Anders, I like to laugh a lot, and most people are just too serious. My aunt used to say, 'We all have to get old, but we don't have to get older.'"

*

After I got that surprise answer to the question "What's the best part about turning 90?" I decided to ask some of my other oldest patients. I haven't yet been told the classic answer, "No peer pressure," but here are some of the answers I've gotten:

- Getting to look forward to turning 91!
- Just getting up every day.
- The people. Everyone treats me like I'm a celebrity just because I've lived a long time and haven't died yet.
- I can do anything I want and say anything I want.
- I just turned ninety, but I can still drive and go. I have something planned each day. I have a lady friend and she and I see pretty much eye to eye on things. We have a good time.
- I live alone now, so I can do anything I want. I play dominoes with my church friends until late at night, then I sleep until noon if I want.
- Looking younger than I am.
- Nothing!
- I can look back and say, "I made it!" But I really don't spend any time thinking about how old I am.
- I can still play golf, unlike the other sports I love.
- The women don't chase me like they used to.
- I can go to Target or Home Depot, push a cart around the store for exercise, then leave, and nobody bothers me.
- You get a lot of help. People give you help even when you don't feel like you need it. You feel silly, but you accept it...you take advantage of it.
- If you like people, you can make friends with folks of all ages. You can relate to children, and others all the way up

33

to the old people like me.

- I'm living today and looking for tomorrow. I'm not one of those who lives in the past.
- I'll get to go to heaven real soon.

*

Mr. Maple is an 81-year-old man whom I had already seen a few times as a patient. Retired, he was still energetic and engaging, lovingly doting on his wife whose illnesses required more frequent visits to a number of different doctors. He accompanied her to each appointment and learned quite a bit about her conditions and her doctors in the process. A successful businessman, he was a lifelong student. But today, he was the teacher.

"Dr. Anders, good morning. It is always *good* to see you!" His enthusiasm was typical of his approach to life. He exuded friendliness and optimism, which made the contrast with his next statement all the more sharp.

"I don't know if you know Dr. Mort, but don't *ever* send one of your patients to him."

I knew of Dr. Mort — a well-trained and very competent specialist. I knew of no reason not to trust his medical skills. But Mr. Maple continued.

"We had an appointment to see him, and had to wait in the front waiting room for over an hour, and then we went into the exam room and had to wait almost another hour. He came into the room, and never apologized for making us wait. He didn't call my wife by her name. He never looked her once in the eye, just spent all his time typing away at that silly computer."

I knew better than to ask why his wife had to see Dr. Mort or how he had treated her medical condition. To them that no longer mattered. He could have been a Harvard trained, Nobel prizing winning doctor, but that was not how his medical care and

34

skills would be measured.

I am not sure who first said, "People don't care how much you know until they know how much you care," — I've heard it attributed to several different people. I've tried to remember that quote, and I've never been disappointed when I did.

*

Dr. Harry Cheves was the most respected physician (other than my parents) I knew of growing up. He had a general medical practice in East Point, GA alongside my father's obstetrical office, about 30 minutes away from where I currently live and practice. He took care of my aging grandparents, making house calls on them when they could no longer get out of bed, allowing them to die at our home with dignity. He performed my physical exam for entrance into medical school.

Dr. Cheves started practicing medicine alongside his father, whose father had also been a physician. When Dr. Cheves started practice he charged $5 for a house call, and even less for an office visit. His malpractice insurance cost $250 each year when he began, but in his later years, despite never having had a lawsuit or even the threat of a lawsuit against him, his malpractice insurance cost him $15,000 annually. Nevertheless, he practiced until he was almost 80 and retired fifty years to the day from when he had first opened his office.

So imagine how I tightened up a bit when I looked down one morning and saw his name on my list of patients for the day. I knew he had recently retired. The transition into retirement can be tough for a man. Men especially receive so much of their identity from their job — it defines them, to themselves and others. I hoped he was adapting well to his well-deserved retirement.

I knew from personal and professional contact just how long he had been practicing medicine, longer than I had been

35

alive. Since his retirement I had already seen several new patients who had been under his care for many years. I felt like I was in an archives museum as I reviewed the medical records we requested on some of these patients. His records of more than 40 years ago were quaint by today's standards, with the single digit fee and progress note all scratched onto a single 4x6 card. His care had been excellent, and every one of his patients I met was sorry to be forced to find a new doctor.

I enjoyed my first appointment with him as his doctor, hoping I could make others feel as relaxed as he made me. We reviewed his health history and some of the medical problems he was having. During the exam I recalled the advice of Dr. Dixon Dunlap, an attending physician I had in medical school, who said, "Always pay attention to the hands. They tell a lot about a man." Dr. Cheves' hands were thick and strong, and he wore a Medical College of Georgia Class of 1953 ring. It was well worn from decades of wear — a sacred relic that defined the wearer.

I decided that perhaps some changes in his treatment were in order, but felt that out of respect for him that rather than making any changes myself, I would first refer him to a neurologist to confirm my impressions. He deserved the V.I.P. treatment, and I thought that he might look upon someone else as being more authoritative than a boy he had watched grow up. As I reviewed my plan with him I couldn't help but continue to notice the well-worn "53" on his ring — all the years of service, all the years of sacrifice, all the years of being 'Dr. Cheves'. He deserved all the respect I could offer, and more. A referral to a specialist would be in keeping with that plan. And so the referral was made, with a return visit to me to follow-up after the specialist had provided his advice.

I saw him back after a few weeks, and started to talk with him about what had been decided with the neurologist. Since I hadn't yet received a letter summarizing the findings of the neurologist, I was curious to hear what Dr. Cheves had to report about what the neurologist thought was the correct diagnosis, what medications he changed, and what additional tests were ordered. But Dr. Cheves didn't start off with that information. When I asked, "How did things go with the neurologist?" he responded with an unexpected reply: "I really didn't care for him. He seemed too busy, too rushed. He didn't listen at all to me like you did — like I did when I was still practicing. He seemed like he wanted to get out of the room almost as soon as he got in."

I felt embarrassed for my colleague, who I knew to be an excellent diagnostician, and yet I was also surprised that Dr. Cheves was offended by the fast paced world of medicine that so many doctors seem to exist in these days. The lower reimbursement rates that insurance companies and Medicare force on doctors leave them with seemingly no other option to protect the bottom line in a world of rising costs due to malpractice insurance, office overhead, and increasing requirements for paperwork that isn't reimbursed. I'm sure I've been in that other doctor's shoes before, and I felt guilty realizing someone might have reason to think that of me. But shouldn't Dr. Cheves of all people understand?

No! Of all people, he had earned the right to say how medicine should be practiced. And so I listened to his critique of modern medicine and tried to learn from him. Later I would refer him to another neurology group, and fortunately he would give glowing praise for the care he received from them. But for now he wanted to talk; he had more to say.

Dr. Cheves continued with his update. "I had to stand between him and the door just to keep him in the room long enough to answer some of my questions. I filled out my long information form completely, but it was as if he had never even looked at it — he asked me most of the same history questions I had already filled out on the form."

His rich southern voice continued to recount the episode and I could tell how deeply this encounter saddened him. But his sorrow seemed not to be directed inward; rather he seemed to mourn for the next generation of physicians, for the next generation of patients, and for the profession to which he had dedicated his life. His voice softened as he concluded his report with, "He called me 'Mister' Cheves."

*

I have been blessed in my career to have been influenced by many good doctors who served as role models. What I learned from them has made me a better physician, and what weaknesses I demonstrate would certainly be lessened if I could only more steadfastly apply what they have demonstrated. I wrote about one such mentor years ago before I entered private practice, but I have drawn on his example in the years since. His equanimity in dealing with a dignified older gentleman impressed me then, and now:

On Speaking a Foreign Language

Dr. Mendez standing, redirected his conversation to the family. His voice was a little softer than during the introduction. Each face in the room became solemn. How odd it seemed to me that even in my senior year of residency training, and despite the fact that my attending physician was discussing a topic with which I was very familiar, I could not understand a word he was saying. An occasional word sounded familiar, but otherwise phrases flew by. What I could glean from the conversation was based on Dr. Mendez's posture, the serious yet soothing tone of his voice, the look on his face. I felt a bit out of place and remembered how the day had started.

"Before we make rounds on our regular

38

patients this morning, I have one other patient we need to go by and see first." Our attending physician, Dr. Mendez, continued by giving a brief history of Mr. Amaya. He was a retired executive who had come to him from their mutual birthplace, Puerto Rico, for a second opinion concerning recent abdominal swelling. A CT scan of the abdomen, done the day before, had confirmed the previous diagnosis of a diffusely metastatic malignancy.

Since none of the housestaff on the team spoke Spanish, we would simply be observers during Mr. Amaya's brief hospitalization. As we walked to his hospital room, I listened to Dr. Mendez talk but I realized that I was listening less to what he said than to how he said it. His English was smooth, with well-selected words and only an occasional accent. I was suddenly very curious to watch and hear him interact in his first language.

We entered the room with a single bed, where we found Mr. and Mrs. Amaya and their son. Mr. Amaya, a well-groomed, fit-appearing gentleman about 65 years old, had an alert eye. His smile was pleasant, but his eyes telegraphed his concern. He wore silk pajamas and robe and sat in a chair beside the bed. As Dr. Mendez spoke briefly to Mr. Amaya in Spanish, my sophomore year in high school, when I had droned "Buenos dias, Buenos tardes, Buenos noches," seemed like centuries ago. Dr. Mendez then turned to the ward team and introduced us to Mr. and Mrs. Amaya and their son. We exchanged pleasant smiles and nods, each realizing that more important things were to be discussed.

And now Dr. Mendez was discussing his

findings with Mr. Amaya and his family. Periodically, his wife or son would nod or ask a brief question, but I realized that for them, Dr. Mendez was probably also speaking a foreign language. How could they fully understand the deep meanings and implications of "maligno" or "metastasico" while their minds raced with fear through the eventualities of this inevitable death"? Were they, like me, taking in this conversation mostly by observing the way Dr. Mendez stood, by the tone of his voice, by his obvious willingness to try to explain and offer comfort and compassion in a terminal situation? Had I yet developed the same skills in communication? Could I convey empathy as effectively as "hard facts"?

We left the room in silence. Once in the hall, Dr. Mendez turned to the intern and said, "We'll go next to the new patient admitted last evening. Tell me about him as we walk."

Our team started down the hall while the intern began, "Mr. Burns is a 29-year-old homosexual male with a three-week history of a non-productive cough..."

*

A great example of a loving servant is the caretaker, quite often the daughter or daughter-in-law, who provides care to elderly parents. Growing up I saw my mother act as the primary caretaker of my father's elderly aunt who lived with us for seven years as she was overcome by arthritis and Alzheimer's Disease. My mother made her service seem so natural a part of her life and of our family that it never occurred to me that things could be any other way.

Now my mother and father live with us, and my wife, Kenya, is the example of a loving servant. Her actions silently speak volumes about her values and character. Both of my parents are still fairly independent, but Kenya finds a way to help out. She does their pedicures, cuts his hair and trims his beard, and drives him to church each Sunday in a separate car so he can come home early (since sitting through the complete services causes him to experience too much arthritic pain). She magically fills their vases with freshly-cut roses and mums, and just as magically fills their dishwasher or empties their garbage. Fresh-baked bread or hot meals appear regularly. The birdfeeder out their window has a bottomless supply of seed in it, and their fountain and patio that looks out over Lake Kedron is always picturesque with in-season plantings. She does all this and much more in what she would never call a sacrifice, but would describe as a message of love, for them and for me. She seems to have a burden for their needs. Amazingly, she does it in her "spare time", because she is also the mother for our five children and works daily as a dermatologist.

In this regard, my wife is special, but statistics would say not unique. Across the country daughters and daughters-in-law are providing a massive amount of elder-care for those elderly who are healthy enough to otherwise live in the home setting.

As you read at the opening of this book, this book is dedicated to Kenya and thus to all the others who serve similarly, for she represents the love that is given to the elderly by family members across our country.

At our wedding Kenya quoted the words of Ruth to her mother-in-law, Naomi:

> *"Entreat me not to leave thee, or to return from following after thee: for whither thou goest, I will go; and where thou lodgest, I will lodge: thy people shall be my people, and thy God my God." (KJV)*

How little did I realize then what a Ruth I was getting for my Naomi.

*

Occasionally, I meet someone whose spouse, now departed, is missed, but the surviving spouse implies or frankly admits that there were some rough waves during their voyage of marriage. Mrs. Davidson was one such widow when describing her easily irritated husband.

"He was not a very optimistic person — he was happy as long as he was miserable. He was a bit of a curmudgeon." But she seemed to have adapted to his personality, balancing it with her obvious optimism. "Too many people get divorced," she said, as if to answer my thoughts about what had been the attraction that brought and kept them together. "Being human isn't a crime. That isn't a reason to divorce someone."

*

The loss of a spouse affects different people in different ways. I am encouraged to see that over time the sense of loss often fades some and is overgrown by gratitude. There is usually an attitude of gratefulness to realize the years of joy that were spent with the now departed spouse. With this realization can come a new appreciation for relationships with family, a new understanding for how important it is to be a committed partner to guarantee a successful marriage, and a desire to spread this message to anyone lucky enough to still have an opportunity to improve their marriage before time takes it away. Mr. King was one such survivor.

He had lost his wife of many years to a slowly progressive disease, and had cared for her unfailingly to the end. I didn't meet him until after her death, but immediately admired the intensity and enthusiasm he still had for life, despite the recent tragedy he had lived. On his second or third visit, his intensity was as evident as ever as he started our visit. "Doctor, I'm almost eighty years old. I don't plan to ever remarry. But I think anyone who is married, or is going to be married, needs to read a copy of 'Dear John'. People seem to have forgotten how precious marriage is, and there are just too many divorces. Will you give me a copy so I can send copies to some folks I know?"

"Dear John" is an essay I wrote that was published in the Journal of the American Medical Association in 1988. At the time I was hopeful that my writing it might somehow catch the attention of a doctor reading the journal who might be considering divorce. I have a copy of it hanging above the water fountain in my office and am always pleased to give a copy to any patient who asks. I hope it also enriches your perspective:

Dear John,

Kenya and I had dinner with Lisa last night. She seems to be making the adjustment to being a single parent fairly well. Some people may think I'm crazy to be writing you this letter, but I have my reasons. You and I have always understood each other – more like brothers really – as we went through grade school and high school and being roommates at college and medical school. I never told you that one of the greatest honors in my life was being best man when you married Lisa. But things change.

I recently read that 1,187,000 couples were divorced in 1985. Why does divorce have to happen? I don't suppose those 1,187,000 couples understand why. I don't imagine you understand why. I don't understand why. I guess it's too late to do much for the "Class of 1985", but if those currently considering divorce could talk with you or with Lisa I wonder if they wouldn't give it another chance.

As I said, Lisa is doing OK. She has become fiercely independent in some ways – learned how to paint the house, strip the oak floors, buy a car. Coping in other areas may take more time than the four years she has had to learn: PTA meetings alone, the dating scene, and Will's birthdays...

It seems like just last week that I was on call as a house officer when you called so late at night to tell me about your brand-new baby. Like most 4-year-olds, Will now encounters new experiences with almost every step he takes. I took him to his first football game a few weeks ago. It was just your basic high school game to me, between two teams I knew very little about, but for Will it was a life event — his first exposure to the idea of Musketeers vs. Wild Cats, marching bands, cheerleaders, banners, pom-poms, school colors, kickoffs, and field goals. And last night at dinner I kept him entertained while Kenya and Lisa talked. He asked me if I would be his daddy — but he deserves better than me. He deserves you.

But then there are a lot of kids who deserve better, more than just a father on the weekends. It's ironic that the hard work and long hours that so many fathers invest so their children will "have things better" actually wind up taking away from quality family time at best — or result in parents who no longer feel a reason or desire to be married to each other at worst. And the casualties of the parents' wars are the Innocents.

Seeing what you have lost has made my marriage with Kenya seem all the more treasured. John, I wish there were some way, any way I could

44

get you and Lisa and Will back together – you know I would. But I can't. What happened in Beirut can never be changed. Fortunately for those of us left here, some things can.

We all miss you,

David

(John Rice Hudson, M.D., was assigned to care for the US Marines stationed in Beirut, Lebanon, at the time of the bombing of the military barracks there on October 23, 1983. He is survived by his widow, Lisa, and his son, Will.)

*

Life does go on after the death of a spouse, and sometimes some pretty amazing things happen. I guess we shouldn't be surprised when someone well into their 80's remarries. I know I've learned long ago to expect love to grow where there is soil. Who marries whom can be fun to watch, because some fairly storybook things can happen.

In 1987 my wife and I had the experience of a lifetime. We went behind the Iron Curtain into Moscow and Leningrad as chaperones for a group of high school students. The trip was an upfront look at a part of the world and a culture that I had only heard of prior to that time. When I came home I had a hard time spending anything more than a few minutes trying to tell someone else what the trip was like, but my wife and I could talk about even the smallest details almost endlessly because we had experienced the trip together. For those who didn't make the trip, sometimes the best I could do was say, "You just had to be there!"

There is something truly special about our experiences in life that are shared with others. Those experiences seem more alive when we can reminisce with someone who has had the same or similar experiences.

It is that character of "sameness" that oftentimes seems to lead to some surprising couplings when older adults marry. I have had patients who married an old high school classmate or sweetheart fifty years after both had married someone else, then both wound up widowed, only to finally marry each other. I've also seen a man, after burying his first wife of many years, marry his wife's sister, his former sister-in-law, or his wife's lifelong best friend, or a longstanding neighbor. In no case did I sense there had been any unfaithfulness or even attraction while each was married to someone else, but when both became single again, the shared experiences of the past seemed to enhance the present, making those bygone places, events, and even people seem alive once more. The shared losses made the days ahead seem all the more precious.

I've never been to the wedding of such a couple, but if I did, I'm sure the old Steve Lawrence song, *If It Takes Forever,* would float through my memory, but not because these people have been waiting for each other. They were usually perfectly content in their first marriage and have only the greatest respect for each departed spouse. They would not have plotted that course were their hands on the controls of destiny. Yet in every instance I've seen, the new love seems to build on a life's experience of sacrificial love, smelted by the pain of the loss of a loved spouse, and now reborn for another opportunity to enjoy a life of experiences with someone who has been there all along.

*

The important question is not how old are you, but how are you old?
- Art Linkletter in a speech given at the age of 93

46

Selah
***

Everyone wants to live a long time, but no one wants to be old.
- Benjamin Franklin (1706-1790)

*

The word "Selah" appears in the Bible as an instruction to the reader in the Psalms. It has been said that Selah may be the most difficult word in the Hebrew Bible to translate. When inserted into the Psalm it apparently instructed the reader to "stop and listen", to pause and take some extra time to absorb what had been said.

Many times during an encounter with a patient I feel I should do the same, for a number of different reasons — sometimes to allow the message to reverberate its importance into my memory, sometimes out of respect for the situation the patient is facing, sometimes because additional words simply are inadequate at that time, and sometimes to allow me to be thankful for my circumstances.

In the following, I say "Selah".

*

He's always been ready to die, but nobody's prepared him for getting old.
- Franklin Graham, on the event of his father Billy Graham's 90th birthday.

*

Mr. Cook was one of the first patients I got to know in the out-patient clinic that I worked in as part of my Internal Medicine residency training in Atlanta. As he had aged and been slowed down by emphysema and heart disease he had moved into a retirement home. Modern medicine was unable to undo the damage that years of cigarette smoking had done to his heart. Because his emphysema was so severe, he was not considered a candidate for surgery to correct the blockages in his coronary arteries that were causing him to have recurrent chest pains with any significant physical exertion. So he used nitroglycerin pills if he had a pain, sometimes popping several pills a day.

A lifelong musician, his great love was to play the piano. His arrival at the retirement center had been welcomed by all. He would sit at the piano and play songs that the residents there could remember from the days of their youth — musical therapy for the audience and the performer. Tears welled in his eyes the first time he told me about his piano playing, because he had quit doing so. His cardiologist had advised him that this activity was too strenuous for his heart, as evidenced by the occasional nitroglycerin tablet that he would have to stop and take while playing his beloved piano. He seemed resigned to the advice of his cardiologist, but he missed his music.

As a trombonist, I could understand his sadness. We have all heard about the "runner's high" that athletes experience with the release of endorphins while exercising. I have long believed that musicians (and perhaps their listening audience) experience a similar phenomenon during a performance. To deprive him of the opportunity to play for himself and others seemed cruel. So he and I discussed his life, and we both agreed that if he died while playing the piano, that was not such a bad way to go.

He resumed playing the piano. I never saw him cry again.

When he died 18 months later, I was glad that his final days were spent doing what he enjoyed, and that death for him had come relatively quickly — from pneumonia, a complication of his subsequently diagnosed lung cancer.

*

There is certainly a higher probability that medical problems will impact a person more negatively as they get older and older. Mr. Brady was 94 years old. I had seen him several times before and on his best days he was sometimes crusty and a bit cynical. He had recently had a heart attack and required an oxygen pack to help fight his emphysema. He was now seeing me as a work-in appointment because he had fallen the night before. My staff created an appointment slot that did not exist at the end of a long day so he could be seen, fearing the pain he was having after his fall could be a fracture.

He had several bruises on his shins and hands from his recent fall. Fortunately, there did not appear to be any broken bones. He seemed a bit disappointed in himself for having fallen. While having a somewhat cynical personality type, his view of the world had never previously impacted on his view of himself. Today something seemed different. "This (expletive) old age is for the birds. Virtue is its own reward, and so is old age!"

I thought perhaps he was trying to be funny, but at his stage in life depression and other underlying problems can be overlooked as the patient and doctor simply attribute everything to "old age". If he was trying to tell me something, I needed to listen. So I downshifted a gear, slowing down to take some extra time with him. We talked about several areas of his life, his frustrations, his loneliness, his fears. Along the way I pointed out how many people I knew were concerned about him, supported him, loved him: the staff at his assisted living facility, his family, even my staff, which I pointed out (for emphasis) was now staying overtime to help me help him, and doing so without complaint. (Selfishly, I'll also admit that I was also thinking to myself that their overtime was costing me "time and a half" on the payroll, something I don't like to have to do. Medicare does not consider that a reasonable expense.) As he left, I hoped the changes I had made in his care plan would benefit him, but that's not always possible.

Several days later as I was going through the day's mail on my desk I saw a hand-addressed envelope with large, wavering writing. I opened it to find a Snoopy card that read, "For service above and beyond the call of duty...Thanks". More important to me was the message Mr. Brady had written inside, "Dr. Anders, I want to express my appreciation for you seeing me after-hours." I was humbled to realize the extra effort he had gone to in voicing his appreciation, a response that seemed more charitable than had been my concerns on the day I had seen him. I could never have guessed he would demonstrate such a kind gesture. The rarity of such an acknowledgment is one of the reasons that I have kept this card.

*

To this day, I'm not sure if the man who told me the following was making a joke or a poignant observation.

He was recently retired and wanted a checkup. Apparently he had done a great job planning for his retirement, giving the impression of being financially comfortable and confident.

Unfortunately for him, his retirement planning had not taken into consideration his health. He was starting to pay the price for years of self-neglect — obesity and smoking had led to little energy, diabetes, hypertension and lots of arthritic pain. He was by no means disabled — yet — but he certainly felt every year of the sixty-six he had lived.

After the exam, we discussed his emotional state. We reviewed my findings and impressions, the necessary diagnostic testing I would order to confirm my suspicions and rule-out some others, and what he could do. More than once in our discussion the association between his life style, his choices, and his current state of health seemed to come up. I think he wanted me to tell him he was just getting old, and he had to accept his problems as simply being due to "old age". But I wasn't willing to let him off the hook without at least having him accept some responsibility for his condition, with the hope that he would also accept responsibility for changing his habits and improving his future condition. I encouraged him with my observations that successful weight loss can be a real fountain of youth. I am repeatedly amazed by how improved, how much younger people in his condition feel when they lose weight (and quit smoking!). At the age of 66 years, he had the prospects for a full and rewarding retirement ahead of him, if he would just take advantage of the opportunities.

When I concluded, he paused, and I was hoping maybe he was hearing what I had to say, and accepting it with encouragement. But his eyes didn't reflect much change. "Doctor Anders, you've heard it said that, 'Youth is wasted on the young', but I'm here to tell you that, 'Retirement is wasted on the elderly'."

*

The average octogenarian knows of more people who are dead than living. Think about just what that would be like. You

51

become the oldest person in your family, meaning all your grandparents, aunts, uncles, parents, and most, if not all, of the people you knew growing up and even in early adulthood — siblings, classmates, close friends — have died. One of the great tolls of living a very long life is this process of having to watch so many of your loved ones die. This sobering realization can be burdensome to even the most optimistic survivor. "I've stayed at the dance too long," remarked an elderly but healthy woman reflecting that almost all of her friends have died.

*

One common feature for many of my older patients is that they have family members who have also lived for a long time. Longevity does seem to have a genetic basis. I often ask my older patients how long the oldest member of their family lived. Mr. Pemberton was a spry 85-year-old man who seemed as though he would easily live to be 100 years old. I asked him if he had any one in his family tree who had lived to be 100 and he responded, "I want to go for the family record — my great-grandfather lived to be 103 years old." He spontaneously added, "I remember when I was 15 years old and he had just turned 90, I asked him if he ever thought about death, and he told me he had. He said he thought about how long you stay dead."

*

We all do things to try to make ourselves look better, to make ourselves look younger. When I examine an older patient I sometimes find myself wondering what will I look like when I'm older? How will my hands change? What will happen to my hair? What will my skin look like? Will I age gracefully, or suddenly? What is it like to look in a mirror, remembering or even expecting to see the face you had when you were twenty, only to be surprised to see a face that looks older than you remember your own grandfather? How do we come to terms with the daily reminder of our own mortality?

One patient confided similar concerns about her own appearance and admitted to comparing herself to others. She was walking down the street one day, thankful not to be the little old lady she could see hobbling down the sidewalk across the street from her. Imagine her surprise when, as she said, "I finally looked directly over to the woman, who was no longer there. I was looking at a large storefront plate window, seeing my own reflection."

*

Mr. Patel was a man from India who was older than seventy when I first met him. Seeing his small, thin, but surprisingly muscular frame the first time I met him, I guessed he hadn't been in our country long, or at least he didn't care very much for our western diet. I was right on both accounts. I enjoyed getting to know him over the next few visits. He told me he had come to live in the U.S. since his children didn't think he would be happy alone after his wife died. He now lived with his older son, but he saw firsthand how busily a high-tech specialist works in the U.S., and in fact the entire family of the son, daughter-in-law, and two teenage grandsons was always on the go. He enjoyed the time he spent with them, but much of his time was spent alone.

The last time I saw him he was planning to return to his country, but hadn't yet discussed it with his son. "In my country, I was happy. I had friends; I knew where to go and what to do. I'm not an invalid. But I'm not happy here. I love my family, but I'm lonely. In my country we have a saying, 'To be lonely is worse than to be in prison'."

I wonder if he is happy now.

*

Mrs. Bell had seen me regularly for more than five years, so I anticipated a routine visit when I entered into the examining room to follow up with her on her blood pressure and cholesterol problems. She had been widowed shortly after I first started treating her, but she had gone on in life and made a new life, on her own, without her husband. She was always a vivacious and enthusiastic woman who just had to sit on the edge of her chair to speak about even the most routine topics.

Today I sensed she was not the same person. I asked her if there was anything she needed, and she said she needed something to help her sleep, but could not finish even that short sentence without starting to cry. As I reached for a tissue she initially waved it off, then took it, dabbing her tears as she explained, "I feel so silly. But my little dog died this week. 'Piddy' was nine years old but had recently slowed down and started losing weight. She was such a wonderful dog — a Cavalier King Charles Spaniel — they are so loving, just what I needed after George died." Her enthusiasm returned as she told me about 'Piddy', so named because she relieved her pity, but also made 'piddy' on the floor — a habit that then continued until she was finally housebroken after two years.

"Piddy would sit at my feet for hours at a time, get up and run to check at the door if she heard a noise, bark if she needed to go out, jump on my lap when I invited her, and sleep on the foot of my bed. I couldn't ask for a better companion."

She continued with her recollections, which I refused to interrupt. Listening to her might be the best therapy I could provide that day. "I took her to the vet, but there was nothing he could do. She developed a cancer on her liver, in her bones... it was terrible. The vet put her to sleep Tuesday." She punctuated the end of the sentence with an inflection that more needed to be said, but silence filled the room for a moment. "It hurt so much when George died, I didn't see how I would go on. Then that dog changed everything. I feel so silly," she repeated, "because I miss Piddy more than I miss George."

*

The shock of losing a spouse, the reality of losing a spouse, impacts different people in different ways. One woman who was in the office for the first time since her husband had died seemed to be managing her grief fairly well. She acknowledged she had a great support system with friends and family all close by, all doting over her. She related her surprise when she realized, "They all love me, but they have their lives, their families. For the first time that I can recall, I don't have someone who loves me the most, who loves me first."

*

It's sad to say, but sometimes doctors just give up trying to help a patient. I suppose sometimes they quit out of frustration, saving their lectures for someone who will listen. But when we as physicians listen, sometimes we become better helpers.

Mr. Thomas came to me as an overweight diabetic. Not just overweight, but a good 100 pounds heavier than the recommended weight for a man his height. His diabetes was requiring more and more oral medication to control, and yet was not adequately controlled. It was time to start insulin injections, but I felt a little frustrated that after several office visits and repeated advice to lose weight, he had never done so, not even a little bit. Now, with insulin about to change his life, I felt the need to dig deeper, to motivate him to take control of his diet, rather than just give up and use insulin. So I told him that I did not see any effort on his part to lose weight. I wanted to know if he was interested in having better health. His reply started with an excuse I've often heard, "Well doctor, I've lived a good life and...", during which times patients sound as if they see no benefit in trying to reverse years of unhealthy lifestyles, figuring that the end is near and there is nothing to be gained from suffering with a disciplined lifestyle. But he continued:

"I think we should start the insulin, because I'm not going to be losing any weight or changing my diet. In World War II I spent 23 months in a German POW camp. I saw men die there, starving and freezing to death. When I was liberated I weighed 112 pounds. I can no more make myself suffer by withholding food from myself now than I would cut off my foot."

We talked a lot about his experience, about his life. I agreed with him that insulin was an appropriate choice; he had suffered enough.

*

Aging is bad for you.
- Aubrey de Grey, scientist and aging expert

Memories
***

I tell you the truth, when you were younger you dressed yourself and went where you wanted; but when you are old you will stretch out your hands, and someone else will dress you and lead you where you do not want to go.
- John 21:18 (NIV)

*

When I was a young child I remember how my grandmother would laugh at herself, and at others, while she recited the following poem:

> *I've got used to my arthritis*
> *To my dentures I'm resigned*
> *I can cope with my bifocals,*
> *But — oh, how I miss my mind!*

*

Memory loss is a great concern for many people as they age, the fear of developing a dementia such as Alzheimer's Dementia being greater than the fear of death itself. I am often asked by patients about a lapse in memory they may have had, and I can often reassure them that such an event is actually common and benign.

Mrs. Martin is a 67-year-old lady who was concerned because she had recently lost her keys, something she claimed she had never done when she was younger. She was concerned this meant she was developing Alzheimer's disease. After we talked more and I examined her, I felt confident she was well within the expected level of functioning.

She seemed reassured as I explained, "Mrs. Martin, when we are 15 years old and forget to do something, we are called irresponsible. When we are 30 years old and forget something, we are called distracted. When we are 45 years old and forget something we are called absentminded. Then suddenly when we do the same thing in our 60's, we fear we have Alzheimer's."

Fortunately for Mrs. Martin, her worries were unfounded. For many others, however, the diagnosis is much more devastating, for both the patients and their families.

*

A common pattern today is that the caretaker for many individuals with Alzheimer's disease becomes the next generation, usually the daughter or daughter-in-law, providing care in the home. This new role can be very stressful for a woman who is likely also trying to run a household with children of her own.

I often see these dedicated providers as I am treating their parents and have learned a lot from their examples of strength, devotion, patience, and humor. One daughter confided to me that, "as a teenager I was very critical of all of my mother's rules for me and her sayings, and I swore I would never act that way. But with time as I, too, became a mother, I realized I had become my mother — same rules, same reactions, even said the same things to my son. And now, regrettably, with Mom's Alzheimer's, she's more the child and I'm the parent. So now I've become my mother, and, more recently I've become my mother's mother."

*

Alzheimer's disease is a horrific disease that robs an individual of his very essence and deprives the family of the person they have loved and respected for so many years. One of the great fears of many elderly patients is that they will develop a progressive dementing illness that will leave them unable to care for themselves and make them (in their eyes) a burden to their family. The family does indeed often suffer the loss as the disease progresses, since the family is much more aware of the loss than the patient, who, as the memory loss progresses, is soon unaware that there is a problem. In that regard only, the patient is spared from the disease, but the family's suffering is further intensified. Dementia is a cruel process indeed.

Despite the stress, pressures and sadness that goes with caring for a patient with Alzheimer's, many families do an incredible job continuing to care for patients at home despite their declining health. A balance of love, faith, and humor seems to be necessary to do so successfully, and I am privileged to meet such family members on a continuing basis. The humor that sustains them is sometimes shared with me, such as this story told to me by a woman who was trying to deal with the progressive Alzheimer's of both her mother-in-law and her father-in-law at the same time:

A man returned to his doctor's office for the results of testing that had been done the week before to determine the cause of his declining health. His doctor came into the examining room and did not mince his words.

"Do you want the bad news, or the worst news?" the doctor asked.

"Well doc, I've always tried to tackle life head on, so give me the worst news first," was the patient's reply.

"You have a widely spread cancer for which there is no treatment. Even with the best of medical care I don't expect you will be alive in six months. I'm very sorry."

There was silence, and then the doctor asked, "Do you think you want to know the bad news?"

"Yes," was the reply.

"I hate to tell you that additional testing has also indicated that you have advancing Alzheimer's disease," said the physician.

"Well," the patient said hopefully, "at least it's not cancer!"

*

Mr. and Mrs. Bishop have been married for 65 years. I've been seeing them both as patients for several years, and like many couples, they choose to be seen at the same time in the same room. They appear to have a good and loving relationship, and like most couples they communicate with a combination of techniques. At one appointment, I could sense their conversation was involving more bickering than usual.

She began our discussion.

"Dr. Anders, I'm afraid that Dean is getting hardening of the arteries. His memory is just terrible."

"Oh, it's not so bad," he replied, before I could respond.

"You old man, you don't even know what day it is!" she said, frustrated.

"Yes, I do, it's Tuesday," he retorted, correctly.

"But you don't know if it's this Tuesday or last Tuesday!"

*

Caring for someone with dementia is a series of mundane events punctuated with episodes of frustration, humor, sorrow, anger, disappointment, tragedy and relief. A daughter came into the office one day with both of her demented parents whom she cares for at home, while also operating her household full-time for her children and husband. The daughter had jotted a series of notes to help her remember what to ask me or to report to me, and left the notes with me. The notes were so ordinary and yet illustrative that I've kept them, and reprint them verbatim below:

- *Christmas Day after 1:30 p.m. lunch he went back to bedroom and changed into pajamas, thinking it was bedtime.*
- *Woke up at 2 a.m. on January 8 and dressed for the day. Tried to get Mom up but couldn't. When I told him it was the middle of the night he continued to open the den curtains and insisted on staying up. He slept in his recliner the rest of the night.*
- *On January 9 he forgot to put on his undershirt. When he realized it, he put the undershirt on over his polo shirt.*
- *January 12 — I turned down the covers and sheet on the beds after dinner. I put the decorative pillows in the wrong place on his desk. (I put them in the chair rather than on top of the desk.) He knew something was "off" but he kept insisting the regular sleep pillows were missing from the bed. When I realized he was confused because I put the decorative pillows in the wrong place, I moved them. That settled him down.*

After a thorough discussion, I had also given a prescription for a sleeping pill for him, with proper warning that sleeping pills in the elderly can be a dangerous combination. Most people don't think of sleeping pills as an intoxicant, but they are — after the pill one is "under the influence" and must sleep off the impairment. The risk for confusion and falls is increased in the event of use, even proper use, in an older person. But due to his nighttime antics and the daughter's true need for uninterrupted sleep in order to function properly during the day, we agreed to try sedating him at night. My warnings caused her to be appropriately concerned, so she again returned with notes

61

regarding her attempts to medicate him at night:

Sleeping pill prescription for him:
I put one-half pill in a pill bottle and a small bottled water on his nightstand. I explained it was only to be taken if he couldn't sleep.

- *1st night: Didn't take it*
- *2nd night: Took it before bedtime because he thought he was supposed to (not because he thought he might not be able to sleep).*
- *3rd night: He gave it to my mother after she got out of bed at 9 p.m. and she fell...hitting her head on the wall. She slept until 11:30 the next day. I almost called 911 at 9:30 that next morning but her color was good and she was breathing fine.*
- *4th night: I hid the sleeping pill. If he has trouble sleeping he will have to wake me up and I'll give him a sleeping pill.*

*

But old folks and old oaks
standing tall, just pretend.
I wish I was 18 again.
- I Wish I Was 18 Again, lyrics popularized by George Burns

Faith

***

I've been forgotten by a good God.
- Jeanne Calment on her 120th birthday

*

In conversations with patients, sometimes death and one's own mortality are not so directly addressed, but alluded to. I saw a woman on the day she celebrated her 91st birthday. She was in good spirits and doing well, and as I congratulated her on such a lifetime accomplishment she responded, "But you know, my rainbow is getting a little faded."

Knowing her to be a woman of strong faith and hoping to help her along this reality, I reminded her, "Your rainbow has been longer than most, and I am certain there is a glorious pot of gold at the end of that rainbow." I also reviewed a little meteorology with her, "Rainbows are brightest where the clouds are darkest, and rainbows do fade when the sun brightens." But her life has demonstrated that she already knows that.

*

When I was in college I worked in a hospital to be more certain that my desired future in the medical field would agree with me. I was hired to work as an orderly on the night shift, working the surgical floor. I loved the work experience and exposure to the world of medicine, although I now realize that what I did had more to do with service to others than the practice of medicine. That realization makes me appreciate the nurses who work in hospitals, for they truly do provide continuous service and care that extends beyond medical care, in an environment that becomes more complicated and stressed every year.

Working the night shift in the 1970's wasn't always quite so complicated, and one of my jobs might be to keep an ear out for the "squawk box" that patients used to notify the nursing station when they had a need. Overnight "the box" was usually fairly quiet, but still had to be monitored so the nurses could be notified of what was needed.

One patient on the service was an older lady who had fractured her hip and had it surgically repaired. A few days after surgery she developed a post-operative infection, and then she slowly deteriorated, her body weakened by age and disease, her spirits weakened by the same, neither body nor spirit seeming to respond to all the best of medical care that was devoted to her. The outlook was bleak for anything better than a slow and protracted painful course of incomplete recovery and restitution to her previous state.

One late night in mid-December after all had settled in, the characteristic "ping" sound let me know to go check the box, and the light on the board indicated the call in was from the lady with the fractured hip. "May I help you?" I asked, not knowing to whom I was speaking because her story was unknown to me at the time. "Yes," stated the frail voice in a matter-of-fact tone, "I would like to die for Christmas."

Stunned by this unexpected reply given with no more

64

emotion than one might express in requesting a refill of the ice water pitcher or when asking for an extra pillow, I was scrambling for some reply, any reply, that would provide a degree of comfort. "I'll tell your nurse," was the best I could ad lib.

I looked over to her nurse, who was entering notes into another chart, and she replied, "I'll go," without saying much else.

The nurses did not talk much about the patients they were taking care of, privacy issues and respect being a chief concern. I did feel it appropriate to ask about this patient when the nurse returned, and she assured me that the patient would be OK, she was just down over the ongoing frustrations of not getting better. She was not suicidal, and there was hope for her recovery, it would just take a long time.

I kept an ear out for how she was doing over the next several nights, but there was no change in her condition. I was lucky enough to be able to get a couple of nights off for Christmas, and then went back for another week of work before returning to college. When I saw the nurse taking care of the little lady, I asked how she had done in my absence. "Oh, you weren't here... Just a few hours after we got here on Christmas Eve — so by then it was Christmas — she died."

*

Richie Dzio and I go way back. I saw him get his high school diploma; he held my first born when she was not even a week old, and I watched him lovingly care for his dear wife as she died from cancer. We shared all those things, and more as neighbors, (he lived three houses up the street), attended the same church, and I became his doctor. But we didn't do things in the order I listed. Let me tell you more about him.

He's a delightful man who, in his 80's, is still on staff at our church where he is one of the boldest and most effective speakers for our faith, especially in one-on-one situations, that you will meet. This is his second career; he didn't join the church staff until after he retired. He is a World War II hero, not just for what he did once he was in, but what he did to get into the service. He was medically disqualified, underage, underweight, and (he thought) under height, so he had to finagle his way into the military. He told me he ate bananas "until they were coming out of my ears" to get his weight up to the required 105 lbs. He had to drop out of high school, and then he had to lie about his age. On the way to sign up he stopped by the butcher shop where his brother worked. Richie grabbed onto a meat hook with both hands and suspended himself above the floor while his brother and another friend held onto his legs and pulled down, hard, hanging onto him to try to stretch him out. The stretching out worked, and he added 1/4" to his 5' 1 3/4" height, making himself 5'2", (although he later found the height requirement was only 5'0").

When he arrived at the enlistment center, he held himself back in line, memorizing the eye chart answers he heard those ahead giving. He was blind in one eye as the result of a childhood firecracker accident, and didn't want that to keep him from serving his country.

He was inducted into the army, and was in the Pacific Theater. He contracted malaria, a case so severe he was hospitalized, and yet when he heard he was going to be shipped back to the U.S. for treatment he went AWOL from the hospital and walked 10 miles overnight through enemy-occupied territory to rejoin his unit.

He was there for the liberation of Manila, and recalls, "the only building that wasn't hit was the brewery. It didn't have a single bullet hole. Apparently both sides felt it was too precious to them!" He didn't see his size as a detriment, but rather saw it as an advantage, laughing, "All the bullets flew over my head."

He returned to the states after the war, and had a great and long life with his loving bride, Margaret, and then they retired to

Fayetteville, GA to live happily ever after. But happily ever after ended when she found out she had cancer, and left him far too soon. His newly renewed relationship with God carried him through those dark days, and friends tried to help as they could. My wife took our new daughter, Rebekah, to visit him when she was only a few days old. Who doesn't feel a little cheer by holding a baby?

He determined to use the years he had remaining serving God, and has done so admirably, now well past 85 and still an active member on staff at our church, visiting others regularly, enthusiastically sharing his faith.

When some local educators found out about his life experience and how he dropped out of high school to serve in the war, they encouraged him to apply for his high school diploma. A recent law passed in Georgia allows veterans of his era to be granted a high school diploma. I was fortunate enough to be there at the Fayette County Board of Education meeting to see him receive his diploma from the Superintendent. It was a proud night in his life. His sister, a school teacher, had always encouraged him to earn his diploma, and now he had done so.

Recently Richie has come on bad news, as he, too, was diagnosed with cancer. If he could talk with you, he would ask you to pray. But he wouldn't be asking you to pray for him. He'd just want you to be praying. He's that kind of guy. He knows what prayer has done for him, and he'd want the same for you.

Richie died a few months after I completed this writing... but he'd still want me to tell you to pray.

*

Surrounded by the urgent issues of life — the car needs transmission work, I've got a meeting with the teacher, the computer is getting slower and slower — we may not take the time necessary to consider the important issues of life. We may think

67

there will be time later to sort out the questions we have.

I've heard life described as being similar to standing in a long line at a security check point. When you are in the back of the line you busy yourself with the goings-on around you, passing the time with things other than the screening you are about to undergo. Only when you get to the head of the line do you begin to listen to the instructions, now paying attention to what will be asked of you and expected of you, preparing yourself to make passage through the screening as smooth as possible. But what if we did as Richie Dzio did when he was trying to pass his vision test — what if we started listening earlier so we could benefit from those who go before? How much smoother would our transition through life be if we were concerned sooner, while we are yet far back in line, (although in reality, none of us knows how long the line is for us)?

For the older person, the front of the line is quite visible. Having watched their grandparents, aunts, uncles, and parents die, and usually also siblings, cousins, lifelong friends, and sometimes even their own children, the fact of their own mortality is undeniable and ever present. As a patient explained, "There are no atheists in foxholes, and not many at the nursing home." As we age it is natural to wonder, "What's next?" and I find as my older patients have often become comfortable with their beliefs, they have thus become more comfortable discussing these beliefs.

Hearing my patients discuss their faith, their doubts, their hopes has fortified my own beliefs. With the stories that follow, I hope you will be similarly blessed.

*

Mrs. Bradley is a retired nurse with a spry, energetic enthusiasm for life that is almost childlike in its unadulterated gushing forth. She was trying to tell me how good her life had been, and she said, "Dr. Anders, I am 80 — no, 80 and a half! —

68

years old. As I look back on my life I am convinced of two things. First, I have a guardian angel. I have met her, or him, at least twice in my life, but I've been guarded many other times. And secondly, as I look back I am amazed how blessed I've been. I tried to do the right things when I was starting out, and ever since, and I've been so thrilled to see how my children hold those same values, and now my grandchildren, too. I am so fortunate to be able to stop, look back behind me, and see how richly blessed I am!"

*

"Dr. Anders, I'm really feeling blessed today. Everything is good!"

What a great way to be greeted when entering an exam room — that kind of good fortune could put me out of business! But Mr. Jacobs was doing well, despite his arthritic knees, bad back, diabetes, hearing loss, prostatism, gastroesophageal reflux and hypertension.

As I finished with Mr. Jacobs it struck me that I do often hear similar reports from patients who report, "I am blessed," but usually it is not someone that I would typically envy because of their station in life. I seldom get such an exclamation from my patients who are healthy thirty-somethings. Rather, the proclaimer is far more likely to be over 70 years old, past the age that we think we want to be, yet the intense appreciation for life and its blessings is so much easier, and so much more often expressed. Why don't we share that same appreciation when we are younger? Why do we who have our health, our energy, our family seem to wait until we have lost some or most of it to realize and share with others just how blessed we are?

*

I went quickly back to my office one evening after supper to finish up some chart work that I had abandoned at the end of the day so I could watch my daughter's cross-country meet. With any luck I'd get back home in time for the bedtime routine with my five kids.

There on my desk was a reminder from my nurse that Mrs. Dalton had called after I had left. She "didn't want to bother me," but would I call her in the morning? I knew Mrs. Dalton needed more time than the few seconds that would exist between patients in the morning, so I picked up the phone and entered her number.

Mrs. Dalton had been in my office a few days earlier. The cough that had not cleared with antibiotics had led to a chest x-ray, then a CT scan of her lungs, and then a meeting with her in which I had to tell her she had all the findings of cancer. I had referred her to a lung cancer specialist, and realized that she probably now had some questions.

She answered the phone on the second ring.

We talked for 25 minutes that night. She had been to the specialist, where a biopsy had confirmed the diagnosis. There was evidence of spread of the disease into her lymph nodes, and hope for a cure was smaller than anyone wanted to admit. She said she wasn't afraid to die, but she didn't want to be a burden to her family. We talked about options for therapy, about miracles, about hospice care, about optimism, about hope. She then surprised me and said, "I'm glad I got cancer. Oh, I don't mean I'm glad I'm going to die. But I've had my time. And already this week I've had some great conversations with my daughter. I've always wondered how I would die. I'm glad it wasn't something quick like a car wreck or a heart attack. I'm a lot more thankful for my family." We talked more about cancer, about preparing for death, about optimism, about Hope. I reminded her of her next appointment date, and encouraged her to call anytime. We said goodnight, and I quickly finished my other work.

I got back home in time to help out with bedtime activities

and to say prayers with my children. I prayed silently for Mrs. Dalton, and thanked God for my family.

*

Insomnia, real and perceived, can be a real problem for many of the elderly. As we age, our sleep naturally becomes more disjointed, less deep, and quite different from that seemingly near-death deep sleep we could achieve as children and adolescents. At a geriatrics conference I once heard a speaker suggest that "after the age of eighty, people usually do not spend any one eight hour period of time entirely awake or entirely asleep". As a patient taught me, "Now that I'm old, it is easier to nap, but harder to sleep."

In addition to this natural change, bodily aches and pains, anxiety, depression, and other medical conditions may interfere with sleep. Decreased daytime activity increases the opportunity for daytime naps, which may "spoil the appetite" for nighttime sleep. Further complicating the picture, some patients seem to dream they are awake while they are asleep — they don't realize they have been asleep, and thus worry because they fear they have not had enough sleep.

The challenge for physicians is to know when to medicate insomnia and when to attempt other therapies. Even the best sleeping pills currently available work by making the patient "drunk", and then letting the patient sleep it off. As a result, patients who awaken to go to the bathroom, or get up before the full effect has worn off — one can be impaired and still awake — are at increased risk for falls and the resulting fractures that are so devastating to older patients.

Addiction must also be a concern, even with the newer medications which do seem to have lower addiction risks, but still can serve to "spoil" the patient and diminish the opportunity for a normal sleep process. As I explain to my patients, "normally we

71

have to stand in line and wait our turn to fall asleep. Sometimes the line is fifteen minutes long and sometimes the line is over an hour. But we learn to wait our turn and then when we get to the head of the line, we fall asleep. Taking a sleeping pill allows us to be treated like a V.I.P. — we are suddenly taken to the front of the line and given the next available space. Now, we all like to be treated like a V.I.P., and it doesn't take long for us to get accustomed to this attention. After a while we come to expect this consideration. So we get to the point that we never want to stand in line again. Whether addicted to the pill or not, we still prefer it." So we as patients and physicians must use these medications carefully and wisely.

I have attended conferences where the speaker had given up on trying to talk his patients out of sleeping pills, reporting: "I have learned that I can spend fifteen minutes with a patient reviewing all the non-medical approaches to sleep hygiene, that I can review all the horrible dangers and risks of inappropriately prescribed sleep aids in the elder, I can talk all about falls and addiction, and then after all that the patient will say, 'Are you going to give me the sleeping pill?', or I can just cut to the chase, avoid the ensuing debate, and give them the prescription with a quick warning and save myself fifteen minutes." Hopefully such cynics are rare in the medical profession.

On the other extreme is the physician who lectured, "I refuse to write for sleeping pills. If the patient complains he is not getting enough sleep, I ask if he naps during the day. If he says 'no', then I advise him that he is getting enough sleep, otherwise his body would demand a daytime nap, so he obviously doesn't need a sleeping pill. If he says that he does nap during the day, then I tell him to stop napping, and he'll sleep better at night." Such a simplistic approach may let the doctor sleep better at night, but it doesn't address the needs of the patient, who likely winds up looking for a different doctor.

So we, the doctor and patient, are trapped without a

universally good decision. One lady in particular, however, did teach me something about how to sleep better.

When Mrs. Chastain returned for a follow-up appointment, I asked how she had done with the sleeping pill she had requested to see if she could fall asleep easier. She admitted that it was not the right thing for her, she felt too afraid that she would become addicted, or at least habituated to taking the pill.

"But I found a great alternative," she started.

"Counting sheep?" I joked.

"No," she replied, moving forward with the conversation, not acknowledging the joke. "Remember you told me that with sleep problems, all distractions need to be removed from the bedroom — no TV in bed, no reading in bed, and so forth. 'There are only a couple of things you should do in bed, and sleep is one of them' you said," she remembered, coyly. She did have a sense of humor after all! And she was right — good "sleep hygiene" as the medical profession calls it, requires several steps before just throwing a pill at the problem. The experts always lecture that when there is a problem falling asleep, the bed should be reserved for only sex and sleep. I was glad she had heard what I had to say.

"Well, I realized that the nights I was having problems falling asleep were the nights that I would get in bed and start to review my problems, my worries, my fears, my disappointments...all the 'My, My, My's'... no wonder I couldn't sleep! So I made a new rule. One other thing I can do in bed is pray. As soon as my head touches the pillow, I have to start praying. 'My, My' is no longer allowed."

The thought made sense to me. I've fallen asleep many nights while praying, oftentimes sooner than I'd like to admit. And while I'm confessing my faults, I've fallen asleep praying in church, too! (You know the old joke: "and the preacher said, 'Don't sleep in my church and I won't pray in your bed!'") I was aware of some studies that suggested the brainwaves on the EEG may change during prayer, and it only stands to reason that prayer in bed is relaxing meditation, with potential benefits in several directions. But she continued.

"In my Sunday school class someone shared a way they learned to pray. It is called the A.C.T.S. method, which helps you remember how to pray. The 'A' is for acknowledgment, where we acknowledge who we are praying to, our Father in heaven, the Creator and Designer of the universe , the Father of Abraham, Isaac, Jacob, and Joseph — you see I have learned to go on and on in this section."

"The 'C' is for confession, of our sins. 'T' is for thanksgiving, thanking him for the things we have and experience. And lastly, 'S' is for supplication, or asking for more."

I told her I was aware of this pattern for prayer because of a gifted Sunday school teacher I had once had. I agreed it was a good model to use. She wasn't through, however.

"It is better than good. Some nights I almost hope I can't get to sleep. But when I 'acknowledge', many nights I think about how He is described in the Psalms or hymns, all the glorious things that define Him or make Him unique and I praise Him and tell Him so. I feel such great peace knowing who's in control that I might drift right off. Many nights I do get to confession, and even to thanksgiving. Usually by then my little life and my problems are in better perspective and there just aren't that many things I think I need. So I don't 'supplicate' much for me, but I do for my family, for our president, for the world we live in. And when I wake up at 2:30 or whenever and go to the bathroom, or again at 5 or so, I'll pray again if I can't sleep. I really don't care if I sleep when I pray. One night I prayed for three solid hours. Have you ever prayed for three hours, Dr. Anders?"

I felt guilty to say that I hadn't, although I don't know of anyone else who has.

"Well, it can change your life. And I feel a lot better the next day than if I'd taken one of your old pills!"

Many patients who go to the doctor realize they might have a wait, and so they bring something with them to read, not trusting the antiquated magazines which characterize doctors' offices. I like to see what my patients are reading — mysteries and history seem to be popular — but I am impressed with the number of people, particularly older women, who bring in their Sunday school book and will use the time to prepare for their upcoming church lesson. I usually ask about the lesson for the week, always glad to learn something about scripture. So when I saw Mrs. Thompson with her lesson book, I asked, "What are you studying in Sunday school?"

"We are going over the creation story. I always get something out of going over the story," she said. I nodded a tacit encouragement to continue her thoughts.

"I am getting a better understanding how profound God's explanation of marriage is. In the second chapter of Genesis He says,

Therefore shall a man leave his father and his mother, and shall cleave unto his wife: and they shall be one flesh. (KJV)

"This is a reminder to me of my marriage," she continued. "I've been widowed over fifteen years, but I miss him every day. I didn't know how painful it could be to be a widow. But I guess the Bible warns us. I remember reading this passage as a teen. I was titillated by the subtle wording that implied the marriage act of 'being one flesh'. But when you marry someone and 'cleave' to them you rightly do become one flesh, one being. Which is fine, and how it should be, how God wants it to be. But when one of you dies, that cleaving together — you know that 'cleave' means 'stuck together'; I had a teacher once who said it was like putting wallpaper on a wall — but when one of you dies it means that one of you is torn off of the other. The one who dies is taken away, and the one left has a gaping side of raw flesh remaining, where the skin has been ripped off leaving many exposed nerves that are indescribable, beyond words."

She said this all with a distance in her voice that implied she had thought this over, and made her own conclusions. "So I've gone on, but not without pain. But we do heal, like all of God's creatures, we are designed to heal. Just go for a walk in the woods and look at the shape of the trees. You can tell where they've been broken and scarred, but they heal over and keep growing. What else are they — what else are we — going to do?"

*

We were having a beautiful April day in Georgia, the kind of day that makes it worth bearing the summer heat just to live in an area so beautiful with springtime's azalea and dogwood. I had seen Mrs. Reeves several times, but didn't really recall much about her as I reviewed her chart before entering the room. She was an older widow, and had high blood pressure. We had never had much of a discussion before — she was the quiet type, and I had no reason to expect that to change. We reviewed her unremarkable interim medical history since her last appointment. As we did so I sensed a more pensive tone in her voice, but with her reserved personality I didn't know just what was different.

So I asked, "Is there anything else that needs attention today?"

"My son died on this date 22 years ago."

"I'm sorry," was the best I could reply, momentarily reeling, caught off-guard by how quickly the tone of the day had just changed, how freely she offered the information. The way that she mentioned it implied there was more to be said. Twenty-two years is a long time, except when you measure the death of a child. She was now 82 years old. She would have been 60 when he died, so he was probably 30 to 40 years old. The most out-of-order I see

Nature is when a child dies before a parent, even when the child is an adult. That is a scar that doesn't heal, no matter how much time passes. I do not even try to think that "things will get better" for these parents. For them, life will never be the same, even if they live 100 more years.

I knew that her memories of the boy she had given birth to and raised, the man who had died, must be more painful today. I have learned that my not asking about him would not make things any less painful for her, just as my talking about him could not increase her suffering. The hurting was already maximal, the thought was already omnipresent.

"How did he die?" I asked, hoping to give her an opportunity to tell me something about him, while also realizing that his health history could impact hers.

"He shot himself," she said, flatly, staring at the floor.

I instantly despised this selfish man. How could anyone do such a horrible act? He had condemned her to live the rest of her life, wandering as an empty soul, waiting for a relief that only her own death would bring. Whatever suffering he had experienced was certainly not as much as she had been made to bear in the 22 years that followed.

After the silence that enveloped my attempts to decide what to say next, she continued to speak. She told the story of how her only child married later in life then had money problems which created marriage problems. The marriage ended quickly but the money problems did not (although his parents were helping him out) and he ended his life with a gun. She felt certain her husband, who had "always been a nervous person", had died an early death from grieving over their son and drinking too much, although he could never bring himself to talk about their loss.

Her father-in-law had hung himself when her husband was a boy, she said, using the term "ironically" as she told her story. Medical science would not describe this as irony, but rather, as being predictable. Anxiety and depression are often inherited

77

disorders. Alcoholism is a maladaptive strategy to cope, a form of self-treatment that can only make matters worse. Fortunately, currently available medications make depression a much less deadly disease. Her son, his father, and his grandfather did not benefit from therapy, but maybe she could. So I pried more.

"So how do you cope? How did you go on?"

"You don't cope, you just go on. At first I took medicine for depression, but that didn't change anything for me. I just realized I couldn't bring him back. My eyes don't cry any more. My ophthalmologist says I've used up all my tears. I used to hate spring, with all the painful memories associated with being called by the police, his funeral, the flowers... I got really mad at God. I really let Him have it. And He didn't say anything, which made me think I was right. Then one year in spring, at Easter, I came to realize He didn't have to say anything. He had already spoken."

Her voice became more determined as she continued, "I will never understand God, but that's OK. The entire Bible is full of commands about how we should relate to God: fear God, worship God, love God, praise God. But nowhere does it tell us to *understand* God. So I don't guess we should waste time trying to understand Him at those times that we can't. He knows we can't understand Him. We weren't created to do that. But I have found great comfort realizing that when He wanted to try to explain how much He loves us, how much He cares about us, that He chose to do so by describing His love as, by demonstrating it as, the relationship between a parent and a child. He calls us His children, we call Him 'Father'. A parent's love is the greatest, most unwavering, selfless love we know of, so He explained His love to us in that fashion. And to make things more clear, He sacrificed His Son for our sins. He was willing to lose His child for me," she said with a waver in her voice, but then she added, resolutely, "I don't understand that, but there *must* be a deep love there. I will choose to believe nothing else. If I believe that, I don't need to believe anything else."

*

As any boy who grew up in the South can tell you, Mama always gets the last word. And nowhere should that be more true for my mother than in a discussion of faith. She has been teaching a Sunday school class longer than most people have been alive. When I asked her for her impressions, she passed them on to me with the title, "In Essence", and I am pleased to close out this chapter with her thoughts:

I retired from practicing medicine when I turned 75 years old, but I still receive much pleasure and inspiration from those I know who are in their 80's and beyond. It's just that now they are my friends, not my patients. After living seven dozen years, I should be a Google of wisdom. I'll need to work on that a few more years, but for now, I have a few distilled thoughts to pass along to help younger folks get through the process of aging. First, some random bits of wisdom which I have found helpful throughout the years.

"Don't sweat the small stuff," is advice which Mrs. Nellie Bray passed down. I wish she could have also taught us how to make the biscuits she used to serve for the Men's Breakfasts at our church. She called them "cat head biscuits" because they were BIG. The men liked them that way.

"Be careful what you set your heart upon, for you shall surely have it". I have remembered that from talks in Chapel when I was a student at Wesleyan College in Macon, GA. Our president, Dr. N.C. McPherson, would stir our thoughts with that dynamic sermon at least once a year.

While I was trying to decide the essence of successful aging, I asked several older people what they thought was important for younger people to learn. Rev. Clarence Jett is fairly independent at age 95. He is a retired minister who started in the railroad business and wound up in the pulpit. His age and experience allow him a fairly unique perspective from the pinnacle of his years. He sums up his life this way: *"Knowing that Jesus is my Lord and Savior has meant everything to me. Life is uncertain at best so make sure you make preparations for the next life because it IS coming."*

A friend for many years from church, Gertrude, echoes Rev. Jett's sentiments when she, at 83, says, *"Live each day to give all of yourself to the Lord and to His World. Rest assured that you will receive four-fold in return."*

A lifelong best friend I've had since first grade, Dot, says, *"The happiest days of my life are at the end of the year when I meet with my friend who is my financial adviser and we decide how much I can give away to my favorite Christian causes."*

Rene´, who is well into her eighties but still actively involved with her big family of grown children and their offspring says with her dry humor that she would like to still be able to get them to listen to her instead of to themselves. She would like to tell them: *"Understand the past. Know where you came from. That's the only way the future has any chance because that gives you an understanding of family. Teach children that being kind, compassionate, and caring is the basis for getting along. Be honest and work hard."*

Still more sage advice comes from Betty Jo, a high school friend who now lives in Oregon and stays in touch by e-mail. She writes, *"I think we have it so much easier than our parents or grandparents. Of course, they weren't faced with the technologies of the computer world, or digital TV, etc. But, because we have all these modern 'necessities', we've been able to enjoy so many things that previously were unheard of... My greatest resource in facing these golden years has been my faith. It is my source of strength to meet each day, to find peace in turbulent times, to seek direction for the future, to find fulfillment in efforts I undertake, and to find happiness when I discover friends who share this faith. It is the richest blessing of life at any age and the greatest treasure on earth."*

My husband, Dr. Pat Anders, advises, *"Always be truthful."*

Now, what can I share from my own experiences? After considerable thought and prayer, here is what I would like for those coming after me to know, and how I reached this conclusion.

When I was about to turn eighty my husband and I were invited to down-size and move to a convenient apartment on the terrace level of my son's home. David and his wonderful wife Kenya and their five children now ages 8 to 16 live upstairs. They all enrich our lives and we are blessed to have them. (I hasten to add also, our other five children and 15 grandchildren help us a lot and are included in our many blessings!)

At bedtime the five grandchildren and David and Kenya gather in our apartment for prayers. The children take turns leading and calling on each person to tell what he or she wants to thank God for. Lincoln, the youngest, likes to thank God for "wonderful weather." The older children thank God for good things that have happened. Lloyd often is thankful that God made us a family. Rachel likes to thank God for Annabelle, the beloved family dog. Luke might be thankful for the success of some project his inventive mind thought of. Rebekah Joan is often thankful for success at school. Kenya, rather than complain about a stressful day at work, will be thankful for her job. David briefly, but profoundly, will thank God that He loves us. Pa-Pa Pat is thankful for accomplishing his goals for the day. Grandma Bec will say she is thankful for some happy event of the day. After prayers we say goodnight feeling well blessed and with worries pretty well pushed aside.

I am influenced by the family prayer time and let thanksgiving dominate my own prayer time. It is miraculous the way anxieties fade when I dwell on blessings.

That is essentially what I think is making old age a good time in my life. Things are not like they used to be when I was younger but my awareness of God's blessings makes all of my problems shrink.

And that is the Essence of what I hope those coming after me will hear and heed. At least until I am older and wiser.

Rebekah Yates Anders, M.D.

November, 2008

*

Where is the ultimate limit to human longevity?
Finally, we are able to see that... w »124.0 +183.1×exp(b 2 /
0.0004) (r ^{2} = 0.9395) ... assuming that... (human longevity)
can be predicted to be approximately 124 years.
- Byung Mook Weon, explaining his scientific formula used to
calculate maximum human lifespan in 2004

*

Then the Lord said, "My Spirit will not contend with man forever,
for he is mortal; his days will be a hundred and twenty years.
- Genesis 6:3, ancient manuscript (NIV)

Additional Thoughts

***

When you get older, you count your blessings a lot more... It's a glorious day to take a walk in the park. When you're younger, you say, 'Oh, another day.' I prefer this age much better.
- Tony Bennett at 81 years old

*

     As a physician, it can be an uncomfortable experience to have to try to find some words of encouragement to offer comfort to someone who has just lost a lifelong spouse. In my office I repeatedly see newly widowed women and men, and as a doctor and human I feel it is my responsibility to bring up the matter and express my sorrow and concern. To tell them, "Things will get better," seems trite, even though I know that most things will, although there will forever be a loss. That loss is permanent, and no matter how long the marriage or how chronic the final illness, the appropriate grief that follows cannot simply be medicated away or trivialized by comments such as, "Well at least you had sixty years together."

I have decided instead to validate the survivor's grieving process by making certain they know it is OK to grieve, while I am simultaneously looking out for any inappropriately severe depression. Grief can be a cathartic process which slowly replaces sorrow with thankfulness. So I often ask how long they had been married, and on being told I will respond with something that initially sounds like what they don't need to hear: "Well, research has shown that it does take time to heal from a loss like this, but you will. It just takes time, about one year for every year you were married. So in 53 years, when you are 126 years old, you will be over him."

On most occasions this will elicit a smile, so I'll continue, "But until then, I hope you have some happy memories of your time together to help tide you over during these difficult months." Having broken the ice and being willing to address directly the subject, I then let them direct the conversation into the good memories they have, the problems they are having, or what their needs are. And I continually learn from the examples of strength and faith I see.

*

Most of the time that I am off-schedule in the office and keeping people waiting, it is not my fault... I promise! It is amazing how often a patient shows up in the office, scheduled for one specific thing, and then the "Oh, by the way..." syndrome occurs. "Oh, by the way..." is the opening line for another two or three problems that exist that the patient reports need to be addressed at the same time. Other times I am behind because I could not have anticipated that a patient was going to deserve more time, or, as I might say to the following patients that had to wait, "I'm sorry you had to wait, but one of my patients needed a little extra love today." When a patient's health is being affected due to grief or stress, the stories they need to relate can be fairly complex and long, but if I won't listen to them, who will? If I won't show concern and compassion, who will? And most patients who have to wait are very understanding.

For the rare patient who doesn't seem to understand the realities of trying to schedule the unexpected into a time-based system, I have been tempted to post the following sign at my check-in desk: "We apologize in advance that sometimes Dr. Anders gets behind schedule and keeps people waiting. Thank you for understanding that in order to listen to, diagnose and treat unexpected problems, a rigid schedule is not possible. For your convenience, however, we do keep a list of local physicians who are always on schedule but never give their patients enough time to speak."

When I do take the time to listen, I do a better job of helping the patient, and often times they help me to be a better diagnostician, a better doctor, or a better person.

*

Many years ago I heard a story that has stuck with me over the years. I have been unable to find the story written anywhere, so I regret that I cannot credit the author or retell the story perfectly, but as I recall...:

A speaker was delivering a commencement address to a college graduating class and his advice was simple. "Take care of the old man."

The students were first taken aback, since many of them were still entirely supported by their parents. Now with their sights set on their first real paycheck, the thought of having to start sending money to Dad didn't attract enthusiasm. But the advice that followed seemed more fun to enforce. "Make sure the old man is sleeping enough, make sure he doesn't drink to excess, keep him physically active. His body is more fragile than he thinks, so don't allow him to take unnecessary risks or to be foolish with it." The students warmed to the speaker as he spent his time seeming to lecture the parents in attendance on how to live their lives, prepare for retirement that was just around the corner, love their family, etc. The younger crowd breathed a collective sigh of relief that they were being spared such mandates. Now that college was over, they were ready to be independent, make money and live for today.

They all listened attentively for his final remarks, trying to remember the major points to rub into the sore spots that "the old man" might be feeling after such a listing of responsibilities:

"So take care of the old man. Make certain that the choices you make today are right for the old man. Not the young man you are today, but for the old man *you* will be in sixty years."

*

In his day, Malcolm Forbes was one of America's most wealthy men. For his 70th birthday he flew eight hundred guests from all over the world to Morocco to celebrate with him and Elizabeth Taylor. He had it all, and spent an estimated $2.5 million to have others celebrate with him. So what does one want for one's 70th birthday when price is no object? Shortly before his big party someone asked him what present he would like to have. His response was, "More time." Yet just six months later he would be dead of a heart attack.

I was 32 years old at the time of his death, and was impressed to realize how valuable "more time" is. None of us can ever seem to get enough. Even patients I have known who have lived to be 100 wanted more time. Life is never long enough until pain, disease, or loss intervene. Ironically, the more time we get, the faster it seems to go.

When I was a child my father told me how the years seem to go by faster every year. "It seems like we just finished taking down the Christmas tree and lights, and now it's time to do it again!" he would observe. I had waited an entire year for Christmas to roll around, and it certainly didn't seem like there had been any fewer than exactly 525,600 minutes in the year I had spent awaiting the return of Christmas.

I have come to the conclusion that when it comes to measuring time, we all have one measuring stick and each person's stick is the same length, the length of that individual's life. The stick is just calibrated differently for each person, so that if you are twenty, your stick has twenty notches. When you are eighty, your stick is just as long, but has 80 notches, so the notches are much closer together and it does not take as long to move from one year to the next. When a teenager uses his measuring stick to measure 20 years it seems very long, more than the length of his stick, but when one is 80 years old, 20 years is only a quarter of the length of the measuring stick, and is a much shorter unit of time.

The realization that we all want more time helps me appreciate just how valuable a commodity time is, when measured in terms of what it means for each individual. Time is a limitless pool from which flows a non-renewable resource. Life is precious. Don't waste a single day. Don't wait for your stick to get any longer. It won't.

*

As a physician I have come to understand that we physicians are "Keepers of the Flame". We didn't create the flame that burns within each of us, but we are responsible for tending it.

At times the patient is not able to give a very helpful history, and the physician is required to deduce the facts of the case based only on the findings of the physical exam. I sometimes see things on the exam that make me wish I had a younger doctor or medical student in the room with me so that I could demonstrate some classic findings as teaching points. I remember in particular examining an individual several years ago and the

87

impression it made on me. My observations at the time:

A male, scant hair on otherwise bald head. Does not appear to be in distress, but responds to no commands and is unable to assist in the exam process. Is examined primarily in the recumbent position as motor function is obviously inadequate for walking or even sitting upright unassisted. Pupils equal. Eyes at times will follow an object, at other times seem unaware. Ears and nose without obstruction. Teeth absent, no meaningful speech present although attempts to do so are made repeatedly; salivary secretions accumulate and are more than can be swallowed. Chest, heart, abdomen without remarkable finding. Genitourinary and rectal exam are deferred for the time being, although incontinent of bowel and bladder. Neurologic exam as noted above, with bilateral up going Babinski response. (The Babinski test is a simple bedside maneuver done by stroking the bottom of the patient's foot. If the great toe flexes and curves downward, that's a good sign that the neurologic system is intact. If the toes extend upward in an older patient, that can be an indication of significant neurologic injury due to a stroke, etc. Up-going toes on both sides can indicate an elder patient has had significant injury to both sides of the brain.)

The above patient sounds pretty hopeless, doesn't he? It's not hard to find a patient with similar findings in nursing homes all over our country. We debate about what to do with the flame that is dim and flickering. And sometimes that debate takes on such a tone of objectivity that we seem to lose touch of the fact that we are discussing a human being, a life, an individual who loved and is loved.

So what would you do in such a situation? Do we have enough knowledge, enough wisdom, enough information to make the right decisions? At least sometimes, the answer is no. We simply cannot know all we need to know. You see, the toothless, bald, incontinent "patient" I described above was my son at the age of six weeks, an age when the Babinski response is expected to be present in the still developing nervous system.

It is intuitive for our society to value some helpless individuals by criteria other than those facts currently evident. How do we best care for all of God's creations - at both extremes of age?

*

In the 1960 classic Lerner and Loewe Broadway musical *Camelot*, King Arthur explains that his wizard-mentor Merlyn doesn't age, he lives backwards — "He doesn't age, he just... youthens." Doing so gave Merlyn the ability to warn Arthur about his future.

I have often wondered how life would be different for us all if we all "youthened". But apparently Lerner, Loewe, nor I were the first to contemplate this possibility. Over 100 years ago Mark Twain observed, "Life should begin with age and its privileges and accumulations, and end with youth and its capacity to splendidly enjoy such advantages. If I had been helping the Almighty when he created man, I would have had him begin at the other end, and start human beings with old age. Life would be infinitely happier if we could only be born at the age of eighty and gradually approach eighteen." A similar aging process was depicted in the movie *The Curious Case of Benjamin Button* but in this story an ever-younger man falls in love with a normally aging woman.

I have decided a better plan would be if we all got younger together. Imagine how that might work. We could enter this world old and decrepit at the age of over 100 years, unable to care for even our simplest needs, beginning life in a very dependent state, requiring full care. But over the next few years we would become gradually stronger, more alert, our bodies becoming less ravaged, and before we turned 90 we'd be paying more attention to the opposite sex, fall in love based on the merits we found in another, and get married in our 80's, not so distracted by the physical charms of our lover as can be the case in youth, rather the main attraction being shared values and the enjoyment received from another's company. We'd then spend the next 15 or more years in wedded bliss together without any other responsibility except to enjoy every passing day, all the while spending our retirement fund. When we reached 65 we'd go to work for 40 years or so, enjoying feeling younger every day, as the spouse we married became more attractive, vital, and younger every day.

When we reached 25 we'd leave the work world and simply pursue knowledge, studying the things we found most interesting and important, celebrating 60 years of marriage with the energies of a teenager.

Our life would start to draw to a close as we entered adolescence then childhood as our bodies started to contract into a pain-free and energetic child, then an infant. We would again be no longer able to care for ourselves, although there would be no shortage of others who would want to hold, cuddle and change us for the few years we had left. The stage of our passing would be fairly painless and brief, at worst taking only a few hours, surrounded by the great joy so characteristic of that life event, then we'd wind up as only a twinkle in someone's eye.

*

Sure I'm for helping the elderly. I'm going to be old myself someday.
- Lillian Carter, in her 80s (1898-1983)

Conclusion
***

The longer I live the more beautiful life becomes.
- Frank Lloyd Wright (1869-1959)

*

Looking back, I suppose I could say I first started studying geriatrics when I was five years old. My friend, also named David, lived two houses up the street. One day he took me into his house to meet his visiting grandmother. She was a thin woman who sat in their living room in a chair facing the television, wearing a white sweater although it was summer and in that era no one in the South had air-conditioning in their home. She had a shake I would later come to know as Parkinson's Disease, and she did not say a lot. But she had two luxuries not afforded me: in front of her on the coffee table was a bowl of Raisinettes, and she seemed to be able to watch all the television she wanted, so she appeared to me to be royalty. She also seemed much different than my grandmother. She was... *old.* Not just an adult, but different enough from adults to strike me as being unique.

Later, when I was nine years old, my father's Aunt Blodwyn came to live with us. She was a feisty, stout Pennsylvanian who had helped raise my father, so he returned the favor when age and arthritis began to contract her world. During the ten years she was part of our household she developed dementia which was characterized by confabulation and storytelling of the wildest sorts — the Indians she had just met on the trip to the grocery store with my father, the man who had just asked her to marry him, the requests from someone on the street to go and return to her profession as a nurse. As an adolescent, I found this behavior fascinating, and sometimes I would sit with her in our living room and let her tell me her stories, realizing this seemed to bring her pleasure or comfort that she could find nowhere else.

Meanwhile, my maternal grandparents provided me with another view of aging that was equally instructive. My grandfather could not be idle in retirement and worked as a yardman, taking great pride in the lawns he kept green and trim well into his seventies. My grandmother, featured on the cover of this book, entertained us all with her cooking, laughter, and incredible recall of Bible verses and literature.

They both enjoyed life, and didn't "act old". One Christmas, after they were both well into their seventies, they were late arriving to our house, which frustrated me as a boy since we had to wait to open our packages until they could be there to see the festivities. Grandma was apologetic for keeping me waiting, explaining that Pa-pa had teasingly sprayed her back with a can of aerosol deodorant, and when she shrieked from the cold blast he started chasing her around the room. As a child, I was not sure why that should make them almost a half hour late, but I laughed with her at his friskiness.

They were not immune to aging, however, and came to live with my parents in their later years. He died in my parents' home shortly after I finished college, and she died in their home while I was in my Internal Medicine residency. They were both fortunate that the assistance required by their gradual decline did not exceed the care which my mother could provide for them at home, and our entire family was enriched by their presence in the mainstream of our gatherings and activities.

All along the way I saw the burdens and benefits of aging, able to see that the changes of advancing age are not a disease in and of themselves, although those changes do often predispose to disease. So it should not be surprising that I wanted to know more about this curious phenomenon of aging.

In 1990 I was an Assistant Professor of Medicine at the Medical College of Georgia in Augusta, Georgia. Already board certified in Internal Medicine, I decided to prepare for and sit for the boards to receive added qualifications in Geriatrics. I had no idea at the time that one day I would be in the private practice of Geriatrics in Peachtree City, Georgia, located in the same county I had lived in when I attended high school, and that the area would have so changed, grown, and improved, as to be recognized in 2007 by US News & World Report as one of the top ten cities to retire to. Truly, there could be no better place to locate my practice or my family than right here in Fayette County, Georgia. Over those years my treasured wife and I have been blessed with five wonderful children, my parents are living with us in their own terrace level suite, and I drive one mile to work each day. I am blessed beyond explanation. All of these changes in my life have happened gradually, incrementally, and for the better, much like most of life. Those tragedies which have occurred were unpredicted, and the events I most feared as a child have yet to come to pass, although they are inevitable if I live long enough. So I elect not to waste away what I have today by worrying about what I might not have tomorrow. These are the golden years of my life. I can ask for no more and deserve far less.

I have met some wonderful and fascinating patients during my career. I have had the honor of treating patients who were adults I looked up to when I was a five-year-old boy. I have been humbled to have been entrusted with the medical care for parents of people I went to grade school and high school with, people who sought me out or who were as surprised as I when we made a connection between now and then. I have treated fellow physicians and family members of these physicians. I have cared for four generations of the same family at the same time, not an easy feat since I don't treat children. Some patients' comments have surprised me, while others have given me reason for optimism as I age. And some have done both (like the 92-year-old gentleman who asked for a prescription for Viagra.) Whatever good I have done for them, they have enriched and inspired me so much more.

What true rewards I receive in being a part of patients' lives! Recently I received a card and note from a patient's daughter shortly after her elder mother's tragic stoke, fall, and death:

"Mother was very particular about her doctors — she cared a great deal for you! It seemed every week she would ask me if we were going to see you. When was her next appointment to see you? She would always feel better after her visit to your office. ALL your staff were friendly and caring! I'm thankful that mother had no pain after her fall, and appeared to be so at peace in her coma. The Lord protected her and gave us time to say goodbye. I was with her the entire time and her death was so peaceful. We look forward to the day when we will see her again..."

And I believe we will.

During high school, college and medical school I spent seven different summers performing live entertainment in amusement parks with the Raz'Mataz Dixieland Jazz Band. One thing I learned as a performer was know when to leave the stage, and I think my time is now. As with most shows I was in, I am very appreciative of you, the reader, my audience, and I would love to stay longer. I hope to leave you now feeling the same.

*

If you can make it past 100 you've got it made.
Very few people die after that age.
- George Burns (1896 - 1996)

About the Authors

Dr. David L. Anders is board certified in Internal Medicine and Geriatrics. He and his wife, Kenya, live in Peachtree City, Georgia. They have five children: Rebekah, Lloyd, Luke, Rachel, and Lincoln.

Dr. Rebekah Yates Anders is the mother of six, grandmother of twenty, great-grandmother of twins, and loved by many more. She is a retired physician and lives in Peachtree City, Georgia.

They welcome your comments to them by e-mail at:
Attn: Fred Carey, Executive Assistant
OctoDoc@AndersUSA.com

Or write via U.S. mail at:
David Anders Publishing House
PO Box 2422
Peachtree City, GA 30269

Drop by our website at
www.AndersUSA.com
Find us on Facebook at
David Anders Publishing House

David Anders Publishing House — a Writer's Studio® was established to provide new authors assistance with access to the world of professional publication. As a publisher of quality writings we hope to be adding continuously to our studio of writers and the list of their fine works.

If you have a friend who is trying to get a book published, tell him or her about us — or maybe you are ready to take that step yourself. Visit our website and bookstore at www.AndersUSA.com.

Books we are proud to be featuring currently include:

20/80 A Love Letter...Sort Of
by David L. Anders

This fictional romantic comedy is a story of humor, romance, wisdom and foolishness.

David Patson is a Pre-Med student at the University of Georgia who awakens carefree on his 20th birthday, May 25, 1977, then meets three uninvited strangers who crash his party and take him on what can only be described as the journey of a lifetime.

The Silver Bell
by Rebekah Yates Anders
with illustrations by Rachel Elizabeth Anders

In this short story for children and adults, a young boy demonstrates caring and another view of the love of Christmas is revealed.

Signs of The Times
by Kenya Houghton Anders

By combining familiar traffic signs with valuable scripture verses, students of any age will find learning Bible verses easier and more enjoyable.

You Might Be a Problem Drinker If...
by David L. Anders

Hilarious and yet insightful, more than 100 ways to know if maybe it's time to cut down on the drinking (or increase your life insurance coverage!).

You Might Be a Problem Drinker If... Let's Have Another Round!
by David L. Anders

Picking up where he left off with the first volume in this series, the author provides more than 100 subtle or not so subtle signs that alcohol is causing problems for you or those who nag you.

50724113R00066

Made in the USA
Charleston, SC
01 January 2016